TO HELP BABY GROW STR...
SO DO LOVE A...

FACT ...

Adding rice cereal to the bottle will help a baby sleep through the night.
FICTION! Rice cereal won't help a baby sleep, and it can cause constipation. And *that* may keep baby awake!

You don't have to sterilize bottles and nipples.
FACT! Cleaning bottles and nipples in a standard dishwasher is adequate.

You can't give a baby chilled milk.
FICTION! There is no rule requiring that milk be given warm. Temperature has no impact on milk's digestion.

Soy-based formula doesn't help allergies.
FACT! Up to 50 percent of infants who react to milk protein also react to soy. A standard hypoallergenic formula is the best choice for sensitive babies. The truth? No advantage has been found for using soy-based formula.

Starting solids later will help prevent obesity in life.
FICTION! There's no evidence that early infant feeding practice has any influence on the risk of obesity.

"Babies don't come with an instruction book—but this book is a great start. *First Foods* should be required reading for every new parent! It answers every possible question ever asked about infant feeding and is an easy-to-read, authoritative guide to feeding your infant. A must for every new parent's bookshelf, *First Foods* contains everything you ever wanted to know about infant feeding—but weren't sure who to ask!"
—Bridget Swinney, author of
Healthy Food for Healthy Kids: A Practical and Tasty Guide to Your Child's Nutrition

FIRST FOODS

The Questions, the Facts,
the Answers to Your Child's
Earliest Feeding Dilemmas

BRYAN S. VARTABEDIAN, M.D., F.A.A.P.

St. Martin's Paperbacks

For Mom and Dad

"Vegetarians: A Fact Sheet" on p. 214 reproduced with permission from *AAP News*, Vol. 15, Page(s) 15, Figure: The Vegetarians: A Fact Sheet, Copyright 1999.

FIRST FOODS

Copyright © 2001 by Bryan Vartabedian, M.D.

Cover photograph by Anne Twomey.

ISBN: 0-312-98131-7

Printed in the United States of America

St. Martin's Paperbacks edition/December 2001

10 9 8 7 6 5 4 3 2 1

Acknowledgments

This book would not have been possible without the input and support of a number of people:

- Dan and Simon Green, my agents, for their enthusiastic support of *First Foods* from the moment they saw my proposal. Thanks to my editors at St. Martin's Paperbacks, Joanna Jacobs and Jennifer Weis, who recognized the need for a book like this and patiently addressed all of my issues and questions along the way.
- Doctors Andrea Horvath, James Allison, and David Cotlar, for their review and input to various parts of my book. A special thanks to father and fat expert Dr. Craig Jensen of Houston's USDA Children's Nutrition Research Center for his entertaining and thorough appraisal of the final manuscript.
- Houston's finest pediatric dieticians, Laurie McKay, RD, Shae Robertson, RD, and Holly Jennings, RD, for their ideas at various stages of the book. A special thanks to Suzy Berryman, LD/RD, MS, of the University of Texas Health Science Center for her compulsive review of the final manuscript. Thanks to Judy Hoagatt, OTR, MOT, infant feeding specialist at The Women's Hospital of Texas, for her contributions to issues related to prematures and to Cherie Wilkes, IBCLC, for her review of the breast-feeding material. I'd like to thank Laura Minze for her enthusiastic input in the final hour.
- My office staff at Children's Gastroenterology of Houston—Krista McCamish, RN, Melissa King, Lacy Yeager, and Florinda Hernandez—for knowing exactly when to

page me and, most important, when not to page me. A special thanks to Julie Hoagland, whose impeccable organization of my practice makes it possible for questions to be generated and books to be written.

- My parents, who have supported my writing from the very beginning, even if it did involve a red crayon and wallpaper.

Finally, while I wouldn't generally recommend writing a book while engaged in a busy solo practice, the gift of a loving family makes it possible. This book never would have made it without the support and patience of my wife, Deidre. As a mother and pediatric occupational therapist, your innate understanding of when to push and when to let go help set the tone for *First Foods*. Watching you grow with Nicholas is the one of the greatest learning experiences any pediatrician could ever have.

Contents

Introduction

How did I come to write this book?
As someone who believes in full disclosure, I should probably say that I was terrified bringing my first child, Nicholas, home from the hospital. Like most parents and perhaps you, I was afraid of what I didn't know. And as someone who has a hard enough time organizing my own affairs, the thought of being responsible for someone much smaller than myself was a sobering thought. Despite being a board-certified pediatrician, I knew there was so much I didn't know about the practical day-to-day care of a newborn. I must confess that I shared none of this with my wife, of course, who thought her marriage to me would finally pay off. I couldn't fix cars, repair drywall, or do so many of the other things husbands are good at. But I could care for babies. What I soon learned was that my training at America's largest children's hospital had taught me everything about resuscitating tiny preemies, treating meningitis, and diagnosing heart murmurs but had left me short on how mushy to make rice cereal.

While surviving this transition that new pediatrician parents so often dread, I became sensitive to the same questions and issues that I heard coming up over and over again in my office. I realized that if parents are concerned enough to come to the doctor to ask these questions, it made sense to write a book that answers them. So *First Foods* was born. My expertise in childhood feeding and nutrition has been tempered by my experience as a father, and I think this book is a wonderful result.

In writing this book, being a father and a pediatrician have been equally helpful. As a pediatrician, I learned that parents want rules and guidelines. As a father, I learned that the rules of infant and childhood feeding were not well defined and what rules existed were often broken without consequences.

Perhaps even more important than being a father or pediatrician was being married to and living with a mother. As any good pediatrician will tell you, there are certain questions that only a mother can come up with. While most of my at-home questions were answered without a second thought, I discovered that some questions don't have straight answers. I also learned that there are questions that a pediatrician can't answer until he's been through it.

What's wrong with an all-purpose baby manual?
Nothing, except that the practical issues of feeding and nutrition tend not to get the attention that they deserve. And while most books cover what's normal, they sometimes fall short on what to do when things go wrong. Most books will tell you too much about nutrition and not enough about feeding. *First Foods* will, I hope, tell you just what you need to know. The format of *First Foods* is easy to navigate, and the book is full of interesting facts that you may not find in general child care books. The basic questions are spelled out in bold type so there's no digging to get to the burning issues that you want to know about.

Who is this book for?
This book is for anyone looking for easy-to-understand answers to the most basic questions about feeding babies and toddlers. It's for first-time parents who find themselves changing formulas as frequently as they're changing diapers. It's for veteran parents whose questions were never quite answered the first time around or who find they're dealing with all-new feeding issues with each new baby. Short on theory and full of practical solutions to every parent's feeding and nutrition dilemmas, *First Foods* is for all parents of young children. Whether for the bathroom, bedstand, or coffee table, this nutrition variety book is for any-

one who wants to know the where, how, and why of feeding their child.

How should you use this book?

Enjoy it and thumb through it. This book is organized by age and is broken down into sections based on a child's developmental ability and stage of feeding. It is based on a question-and-answer format and covers the most common questions faced by new parents when talking to their pediatricians. And just to keep things interesting, there are sidebars throughout the book touching on topics related to the questions in that particular section. While you may find that not every feeding issue is covered, the major ones are addressed. Keep *First Foods* close at hand and refer to it when you're unsure of what you're doing. It really isn't meant to be read cover to cover but picked up periodically for reference depending on the age of your child.

Use this book to help you separate myth from reality. Everyone from grandmothers to next-door neighbors have advice on what, when, and how to feed your child. This book will dispel the myths and black market advice from well-intentioned, self-proclaimed parenting experts. If nothing else, share it with the next person who recommends goat's milk for your baby with colic.

Get some sleep. Most questions are too small to warrant a call to the pediatrician but big enough to leave us wondering if we're doing the right thing. Use this book to fill in for those questions and issues that never get asked. As a parent and a pediatrician, I understand that it's those little questions that are sometimes the ones that keep you up at night. And as a new parent, you can use all the sleep you can get.

Why do parents ask so many questions about feeding their child?

According to the *American Academy of Pediatrics Guide to Childhood Nutrition*, parents ask more questions about what and how to feed their child than any other aspect of childhood care. What does this tell us? This tells us that parents are either particularly misinformed about childhood nutrition and feeding or they're obsessed with this part of parenting. Based on my own experience, both are true.

It's easy to understand why parents are misinformed about childhood nutrition. As a developed society, we take for granted the importance of good nutrition. Most of us have never seen, or could imagine, the devastating effects of malnutrition. The attitude seems to be that there has been and always will be enough food. This abundance and variety of food has led to other problems endemic in Western culture, such as heart disease and obesity. Over 50 percent of adults in our country are overweight, and despite our clear understanding of the role diet plays in arteriosclerosis, heart disease continues to be the number-one killer in America. It's easy to understand how a culture that doesn't understand how to feed itself could be misinformed about feeding its children.

Misinformation is only part of the force driving parents to ask so many questions about feeding. Many questions are fueled by fear—one of the most powerful forces that drives parents to do what they do. Parents are often afraid that they're going to do something wrong. While being informed is a good thing, it's important to understand there isn't much that can be done to hurt a child with food. (And what little damage can be done is detailed in the pages ahead, so read on.) Read this book, ask more questions, and follow your gut. In his classic book on child care, Dr. Benjamin Spock himself said, "Trust yourself, you know more than you think you do."

The goal of this book is not to get parents to ask fewer questions but rather to empower you to understand what's happening with your child. If you're reading this book because you feel you can't ask you pediatrician these questions, it's time to find another pediatrician. A book, website, or computer program will never take the place of an intuitive pediatrician who understands not only the child but also the parent asking the question.

Ultimately, the decision about what and how you feed

your child is yours, but you should be informed. Using a book like this to understand one expert's point of view on specific feeding dilemmas is a great starting point. While a little uncertainty is normal and to be expected, consistency and confidence in your methods is ultimately the key to a healthy feeding relationship between you and your child.

THE SWINGING PENDULUM OF FEEDING ADVICE

As much as we'd all like to think that we're smarter than those who came before us, we're not the first generation to address the where, when, why, and how of feeding kids. For better or for worse, recommendations seem to be always changing. It wasn't that long ago that pediatricians were pushing solid food at a month and even more recently that formulas were favored to breast milk. And just as you snicker at the feeding tales woven by your parents and grandparents, one day the laugh will be at your expense by the child in your arms.

While it's a humbling thought to realize that what's here today probably will be gone tomorrow, we can only hope that the future brings even better nutritional advice for our grandchildren and great-grandchildren. It's likely that the future will hold a better understanding of the possible connection between early feeding practice and later disease. And all indications are that the developing brain is sensitive to what's fed or not fed during its formative months. What our children are fed may very well determine the individuals they will one day become. When that day comes, may this book stand testimony to the lunacy of infant and toddler feeding in the early twenty-first century. Until then we'll have to be happy with solids at four months, milk at a year, and the belief that food exists primarily to make our children chubby and happy.

Chapter 1

Baby Basics
(Zero to Four Months)

Despite what you may hear from neighbors and friends, nobody has any idea of what they're doing when they bring a baby home for the first time. It's one of the great conspiracies of modern civilization: Let the first-time parents think they're supposed to have all of the answers. After all, it's instinctive. Well, for those of you who haven't caught on yet, nurturing is natural but knowing how to elicit a great burp takes a little help. And simply understanding and accepting that you're in the dark about some of these things will make the whole process of bringing a baby home less stressful.

Is the stress of having a new baby all about ignorance? No. In fact, most new moms and dads will tell you that their stress comes from the fear that they may do something wrong to hurt their baby. Despite these fears, what few pediatricians and parenting manuals ever tell you is that you can't harm your child with rice cereal or cold formula. At least, it has yet to happen. Even beyond the basics of rice or knowing how formula should feel on your wrist, it's very unlikely that the feeding choices you make will ever cause serious harm to your child. We know from seeing a great many children who have been fed in a number of creative ways that, in most cases, things turn out just fine. For better or worse, concerned new parents are here to stay. And until each parent has reached some level of experience and comfort with that next stage of feeding development, asking questions will be the antidote for parental anxiety.

STARTING OUT

Should I breast-feed or bottle-feed?

How am I going to feed my baby? One of the most important questions you'll answer after you've chosen a name! Next to the influence of your community, partner, doctor, friends, and support network, what should you consider in the breast vs. bottle dilemma?

1. *Be sure to get the facts.* Reading books like this will help dispel the myths that may be influencing this important decision. Consider the pros and cons of breast and bottle, ask reliable sources about what you don't understand, consider your personal circumstances, and decide what will work best for *you* and *your baby*.
2. *Don't decide what to do based on what worked for someone else.* There's no question that to make the right decision, you'll need to ask questions of those around you. Unfortunately, the advice you get about what to do is always biased by the experience of the person giving the advice. This can be good or bad depending on how you think babies should be fed. Remember that the experience you have with your child will, for better or worse, be very different from theirs. This is your decision, not theirs, and in the final analysis you'll never know what works for you until you try.
3. *Be true to yourself.* If you're not interested in breast-feeding your child, don't feel pressured to do it. It doesn't mean you shouldn't try, but don't be afraid to be honest with yourself. If you're doing it for someone else and not your baby, you're just setting yourself up for disappointment when you come to the realization that this may not be for you. Breast-feeding is clearly the feeding choice that requires a greater commitment on your part, and you need to be true to yourself in making this decision.

What's better for baby?

Breast milk is unquestionably the best source of nutrition for babies. Its immunologic properties, digestive ease, and nutritional composition make breast milk superior to formula in all respects. But while breast milk is best for most babies, breast-feeding may not be the best for every family. Consider your baby, family, and personal circumstances when making this important decision and don't feel bad should you decide to formula feed.

Can I change my mind once I've started feeding one way?

If you choose to breast-feed, you can always downshift to bottle-feeding at any point. If you choose to bottle-feed, however, it's much harder, if not impossible, to go from bottle to breast after the first week or so of life. This is one of the strong arguments in favor of giving breast-feeding a try if you're undecided.

Can I both breast- and bottle-feed?

Yes, you can do both, but you'll need to make an early commitment to getting your

Advantages and Disadvantages of Breast and Bottle

BOTTLE-FEEDING

Advantages

- Anyone can be involved with feeding the baby
- Easy transition when starting
- May allow an easier transition back to work/career

Disadvantages

- Cost—a year's supply of standard formula costs about $1,200
- Cost of bottles and nipples
- Time taken to prepare formula

BREAST-FEEDING

Advantages

- It's the best source of nutrition for babies
- Increased maternal weight loss after delivery
- It's free and conveniently packaged—no need for bottles and nipples
- Decreased incidence of diseases in baby
- Improved mother-infant bonding

Disadvantages

- First two to three weeks may be challenging
- Only Mom can feed the baby initially
- May not always be socially convenient
- Some diet restrictions such as alcohol

baby started on breast-feeding before you switch over to bottle-feeding. Whether you plan to express and feed by bottle or simply supplement with formula while at work, the first few weeks will require the same persistence as that of a mother planning to breast-feed exclusively.

What role should Dad have in the feeding decision?

While the decision about whether to breast-feed should belong to the mom, remember to consider the dad's wishes. Despite the family involvement that bottle-feeding allows, many dads have strong feelings about the advantages that breast milk appears to provide to their children. Be sure to ask.

How soon after birth does a baby get her first feeding?

This depends on how you plan to feed your baby and the policy of the hospital where you deliver. Most delivery suites will offer you some time alone with your baby before she's taken to the nursery for routine newborn care. This is a perfect time to put your baby to the breast for the first time. In fact, early feeding may be important since studies have shown that breast-feeding has a higher chance of success if the baby is put to the breast within the first hour of life. If you are unsure about your hospital's policy regarding feeding shortly after birth, be sure to inquire during your predelivery visit. Babies who are not offered their first feed by breast usually will receive their first bottle feed within four hours after delivery.

Why do nurseries offer sugar water to babies before breast milk or formula?

While some nurseries will allow babies to be put to the breast immediately, it's still common practice in many hospitals to provide water at the first feed. While uncommon, abnormalities of the swallowing tube and airway can lead to the aspiration of milk into the lungs. Water is the safest substance to start with in the event that there are unexpected problems.

Can the epidural anesthesia that I received during labor affect the way my baby feeds?

Several studies comparing infants of mothers with and without epidural anesthesia have shown that infants born to mothers with epidurals pick up their feeding more slowly than their drug-free nursery mates. Does this mean that you shouldn't elect to take an epidural? Not necessarily. The differences between babies of mothers with and without epidurals aren't significant enough to warrant a decision on this possibility alone. Do what needs to be done, but remember, some of what you get your baby gets.

When my baby was discharged from the nursery, we were given samples of one of the brand-name formulas. How important is it that my baby use that formula as opposed to other formulas?

While the formula companies would like you to believe that the use of their formula in a hospital nursery represents an endorsement, this usually isn't the case. The decision by a hospital to stock and dispense a particular formula exclusively as their standard formula most often represents effective negotiating and bidding on the part of the formula manufacturer. Stock quantities of the formula in question are provided free or at cost for pediatricians and nurses to dispense. It is common to provide promotional material to new parents, such as diaper bags and rattles, in hopes that the name will stick when tired new parents are faced with a barrage of formula labels at the grocery store.

Remember that despite what you're sent home with, there are other brands that will suit your baby as well as what was given to you in the nursery. Talk to your pediatrician and don't be afraid to consider less costly options.

How often should a newborn be fed?

Full-term newborns typically are fed about every two to two and a half hours (measured from the beginning of one feeding to the beginning of the next), although this can vary from child to child. Babies should be fed on demand (when they seem to be hungry) and not by a rigid schedule. By the time your baby is a month old, you can expect him to feed approximately every three to four hours and one to two times at night. Breast-fed babies generally have 8 full feeds per day with 2 snacks. By three months you may be down to one night-time feeding or, if you're lucky, none at all.

> **How much should baby be eating?**
>
> Every baby is different, and his activity level will determine what happens on a day-to-day basis. Consider these as general guidelines as to how much your child should be eating:
>
> *First days:* 10–14 ounces/day (10 feeds of 1–2 ounces each)
> *1 month:* 18–22 ounces/day
> *2 months:* 20–28 ounces/day (5–8 feeds of 3–4 ounces each)
> *3 months:* 25–35 ounces/day

How long should a baby take to feed?

This can vary tremendously from baby to baby. In general, a newborn should be able to complete two and a half ounces within fifteen to twenty minutes. If your baby is going through a growth spurt, it wouldn't be unusual for her to take three to four ounces inside of seven to ten minutes.

> **Slow Feeders**
>
> When should you be concerned if your baby is a pokey eater? Most newborns should be able to complete their feeds within fifteen to twenty minutes. If your baby takes longer than twenty-five minutes to finish her bottle, you may want to discuss it with your physician. While the problem may be as simple as the wrong nipple choice, it may indicate something more.

How do I know if my baby is getting enough to eat?

Since babies can't speak (in ways we understand), this is a great question and a common source of concern for parents. Most babies will tell you that they've had enough by slowing down their pace of feeding, becoming disinterested, pulling away, or simply falling asleep. For the bottle-fed newborn, this occurs at about two ounces; for the breast-fed infant, at around ten minutes on each side once she knows what she's doing. Breast-fed infants often will require up to forty-five minutes per feed during the first few weeks of life between nibbling and falling asleep. This is entirely normal at first and should speed up with time.

Keep in mind that a baby's feeding volume can vary from feed to feed and depends on level of activity and mood. As a general rule, a baby should be getting about two and a half ounces of formula or milk per pound of body weight each day. Assuming that a baby takes in this much, she should be having 6 to 8 wet diapers per day, which alone is a good indicator that your baby is getting enough.

How do I know when my baby is hungry or just crying for some other reason?

Unfortunately, this book, your pediatrician, and even the Internet can't help you with this one. Every baby is different. In time you'll learn your baby's pattern of communication and be able to discriminate the cry of hunger from the cry of fatigue. If it's been at least two hours since her last feed and she doesn't seem to be consoled by swaddling, a reassuring rock, or a pacifier, try feeding. Rooting, or the natural reflex of a baby to try to latch onto anything within a neck's distance, is another sign of hunger.

Will feeding on demand spoil a baby?

Despite the rigid approach that some parenting pundits preach, feeding a hungry baby on demand will not lead to weak moral character or a pathetic life of needy dependency. Failing to feed a breast-fed child on demand during the first several weeks actually can threaten an infant's health and undermine successful breast-feeding. Bottle-fed babies are no different, although our ability to control the bottle may make us feel that we can somehow control an infant's hunger and need for sustenance.

It's important to understand that there's much more to the feeding ritual than just food. The response to a child's cry for food or any need teaches a baby that she lives in a safe, predictable place where her needs will always be met.

How often should I burp my child?

Most babies do just fine getting burped at the end of their feeding. Be aware, however, that some children swallow air

---

Dr. Spock—Modern Father of Feeding on Demand

Perhaps more than any other parenting figure of the twentieth century, Dr. Benjamin Spock is responsible for popularizing the concept of feeding on demand. With the publication of his famous book *The Common Sense Book of Baby and Child Care* in 1946, parents for the first time felt at ease caring for their children without the rigid schedules that had been laid down by the generations before them. It was a generation stifled by structure that embraced the kinder, gentler approach to rearing children. Spock pushed aside science and fed parents the folksy, practical advice that made his book so famous. Prior to the Spock generation, parents were encouraged to feed their children by the clock. *The Common Sense Book of Baby and Child Care* ushered in an era of permissiveness and gave parents free license to feed their children when hungry. While in his later years Dr. Spock's advice took a dubious turn toward macrobiotics and alternative diets, his attitude and approach to feeding children by demand and not by the clock remains timeless.

---

while feeding and need to be burped every couple of ounces. Look out for irritability, pulling up of the legs, and pulling from the nipple, which may be signs that a burp is in order.

We have a hard time getting our baby to burp. Is there something wrong, or do we need to do things differently?
The important thing to remember about burping a baby is that no two children are alike and what works for one baby may not work for another. A successful burp occurs when the air trapped in the dome of the stomach (fundus) moves near the valve at the entrance of the stomach and escapes. Depending on your baby's stomach, this will require some experimentation to figure out how to get around his or her special anatomic makeup.

A great position for burping a baby involves sitting the baby on your knee leaning in a forward position, chest and belly against the palm of your hand with thumb and index finger supporting the chin. Gentle, rhythmic rubbing or patting of the back then does the trick. If nothing comes of this, try leaning the baby forward further or bringing her to a more upright position—again, every baby's anatomy is different, and you have to experiment to find out what works best.

My baby gets very fussy and anxious when I stop in the middle of a feeding to burp and won't finish the feeding if I do not immediately return the bottle to her. Is it OK for her not to burp in the middle of a feeding?

Not all babies need to be burped in the middle of their feed. While burping is the antidote to swallowed air, some babies are very efficient at eating and don't need frequent burping. In fact, some infants become so upset at the idea of being away from the bottle or breast that their agitation leads to more swallowed air than what they would get from feeding. If, however, during the middle of a feeding you notice fidgety behavior, pulling from the nipple, or drawing up of the knees, this may indicate that your baby has a slight gas buildup and a burp may be in order.

FUNNY FEEDERS

My pediatrician told me that my baby is "tongue-tied." What does this mean and will it affect her ability to feed?

In tongue-tied children, the membrane that connects the tongue to the bottom of the mouth is shorter or tighter than normal. Except in the most severe cases, this does not impact on an infant's ability to feed or develop normal speech.

How much choking is considered normal when a baby is learning to feed?

Babies shouldn't choke when feeding. Of course some occasional sputtering is allowed, but this should be the exception. Choking and coughing with feeds can indicate nervous system problems, congenital abnormalities of the swallowing tube and upper airway, heart disease, or baby heartburn. If you find yourself frequently helping your baby catch his breath or clear his throat, consider these changes:

- Try feeding with a slower-flow nipple. Sometimes higher-flow nipples deliver more milk than the baby can handle.
- Be sure you're feeding in a semiupright position. Babies tend not to feed well when reclined too much.
- If congested, suction the nose with a bulb syringe and saline.

If these simple measures don't improve things, he needs to be evaluated. Talk to your physician about this one and don't wait.

Feeding Gives Us Valuable Clues about a Baby's Well-being

Newborns don't have a lot of ways to tell us when something's up. Problems with eating, sleeping, and going to the bathroom give us valuable clues about a baby's state of well-being. Be suspicious if you find your baby doing something abnormal during her feeds. Only you know your baby's pattern, so you'll be the first to know when something's up. Taking too much, too little, or too long to feed are signs to call your doctor.

What does it mean when a baby suddenly loses interest in feeding?

Disinterest in feeding is always cause for concern. It can indicate something as benign as an approaching tooth to more serious conditions such as meningitis or bacteria in the blood. Call your physician right away if this occurs during two consecutive feedings.

Our daughter is three weeks old and she is a very difficult feeder. She sucks a little bit and then pulls away, arching and turning her head. It seems that just as soon as she is off the nipple, fussing, she wants on again. What am I doing wrong?
This sure sounds like gastroesophageal reflux, the medical term for heartburn. It's a very common problem among infants. Reflux occurs when the contents of the stomach come backward up the swallowing tube, resulting in a spit or wet burp. While in most cases reflux leads to frequent spitting, other times babies won't spit at all and may simply be fussy or difficult feeders.

The arching and pulling away that your baby is doing is a result of the discomfort that develops from irritation of the swallowing tube. Chronic acid exposure from stomach contents passing up where it doesn't belong leads to this irritation. Most children with this degree of feeding difficulty need to be evaluated. If it proves to be reflux, she'll most likely benefit from treatment with medication.

My baby makes lots of slurping and squeaking noises when she feeds. Should I be concerned?

Extra noises like slurping and squeaking usually mean that there is air getting in around the nipple when she sucks. One of the most common reasons for this sort of squeaking is collapse of a nipple that is too soft. The collapsing nipple delivers

---

Nibblers and Dribblers— When to Be Concerned

The following feeding red flags should be evaluated by your pediatrician:

- Baby isn't interested in feeding
- It takes more than twenty-five minutes to finish a bottle
- Frequent pulling and arching from the nipple
- Shortness of breath with feeds
- Sweating with gray coloring around the lips with feeds
- Significant dribbling or drooling of milk
- Frequent choking that requires you to stop feeding
- Milk coming from the nostrils during feeding

---

less milk, and the baby becomes frustrated only to suck harder and squeak more. The end result is lots of swallowed air and a gassy baby. Experiment with firmer nipples or perhaps a different brand. Different brands of nipples tend to deliver milk in slightly different ways.

Nibblers and Dribblers—Why Your Baby May Not Be Feeding Well

- Prematurity
- Improperly sized nipple
- Heartburn due to reflux
- Oral yeast infection (thrush)
- Lousy-tasting formula
- Viral infection of the mouth and swallowing tube
- Difficulty breathing due to heart or lung disease

The breast-fed baby with noisy feeding most likely has a poor latch, or grip, on the nipple. The characteristics of a mother's nipple or positioning during feed can affect the way a baby latches onto the breast. Evaluation by a lactation consultant should be able to fix the problem. Be absolutely sure to get this one checked out.

Poor latch can lead to sore, cracked nipples, which may potentially undermine your ability to breast-feed your child.

My ten-week-old son has recently become a voracious feeder. He's taking 4 ounces every 2 hours, and it seems like he can't get the formula in fast enough. Is it normal for a baby to feed this much?
Your child is most likely going through a growth spurt. During growth spurts a baby's metabolic demand increases for three to four days, making them appear starved for calories. Consequently, babies will typically take in larger quantities of milk more frequently. Growth spurts are one of the reasons that rigid schedules don't work with babies.

I've recently noticed sweat forming on the forehead of my five-week-old during feeding. Is this anything to be concerned about?
While perspiration during feeding may be a consequence of something as simple as overwrapping or fever, it can indicate more serious problems. Heart problems in babies sometimes will cause children to perspire or become clammy and gray during feeds. Other symptoms of cardiac problems in babies include shortness of breath while feeding, irritability when lying flat, rapid breathing, and blue hands and feet. Your doctor should be notified immediately if your baby develops any of these symptoms.

EATING AND SLEEPING

I have a friend who tells me that I need to get my baby on a schedule and suggested *parent-directed feeding*. What is parent-directed feeding?
Parent-directed feeding is the method recommended in the book *Babywise* of establishing predictable infant feeding and sleeping patterns. It suggests that the early initiation of

a controlled feeding schedule will lead to a happier baby who not only sleeps through the night but understands his role in the bigger picture of family and society. This method of "infant management" has strong appeal for those parents who feel out of control with their new baby or those who want to implement an early element of discipline in their child's life.

Below the surface, parent-directed feeding is a method that's more about parental issues than it is about baby issues. The authors sum up the general mood of this book when they say, "With parent-directed feeding, your baby wins the ribbon of confidence knowing you are indeed in control." Unfortunately, feeding can't be about control. While discipline and relative structure should govern most aspects of a child's life from early on, a child's metabolic needs will vary from day to day and week to week. While regimented programs may make sense from a social and cultural perspective, schedules and an obsession with control don't make sense from a biological perspective. Babies don't need PalmPilots; otherwise they would have been born with them.

My baby sometimes goes four hours without waking to feed. Should he be woken up every two to three hours to be fed?
Most babies will do a good job of regulating their diets on their own. The amount of time that babies go between feedings depends on the capacity of their stomachs. The smaller stomachs of newborns can hold only enough to keep them happy for two to three hours, while two-month-olds can easily hold enough milk to satisfy them for four hours or so. Sleepy newborns may, however, need to be awoken to be reminded to feed during the first three to four weeks. This is especially important for the breast-feeding mother who is dependent on the stimulation of frequent feeding to support her milk supply.

Beginning around two months of age, you may notice that your baby will start to drop her middle-of-the-night

---

Schedules—Don't Worry

Put your day planner away until he's a little closer to a year. Most babies can't stick to a tight schedule as most mothers (especially working mothers) would like to believe. Feeding a baby when he's not hungry and making him wait until after he's ready sends the wrong signal and goes against what his body needs. Let your baby feed on his own terms. In time he'll have his own schedule that you'll be able to predict and work around.

---

feed. In this case it's not necessary to arouse her to feed. In fact, this may represent the early beginnings of sleeping through the night

My child is currently being evaluated by our pediatrician for difficult feeding. She's a very fidgety feeder and takes up to forty minutes to finish a three-ounce bottle. We have noticed, however, that she seems to feed best when half asleep. What does this mean?
Successful feeding while partially asleep may indicate that the baby is uncomfortable during feeding. When going into or coming out of sleep, the baby may not be as aware of her discomfort and may feed better. This can occur sometimes in babies with severe gastroesophageal reflux (heartburn). Reflux causes irritation of the lining of the swallowing tube, resulting in pain with swallowing. Children with reflux often release the nipple and arch as if uncomfortable swallowing.

How soon after feeding is it safe to put a baby in his crib?
Once fed and burped, a baby should be able to be placed in her crib without concern. Babies, of course, should be placed on their backs to sleep since belly positioning has been associated with a slightly higher incidence of sudden infant death syndrome (SIDS).

At what age should a baby begin to sleep through the night?
It depends on your definition of a night. It's amazing the number of exhausted, desperate parents who consider a five-hour stretch of sleep "sleeping through the night." Most ba-

bies will begin to sleep for six- to eight-hour stretches around three months.

Is it possible that a baby could sleep better after changing formula?

As strange as this sounds, it could be possible. Recent studies have found that the protein composition of babies' nutrition may impact

> **Fact or Fiction: Adding Rice Cereal to the Bottle Will Help a Baby Sleep Through the Night**
>
> Fiction. The addition of cereal to an infant's nighttime bottle is unlikely to stretch out the interval between feeds, and it probably won't make any significant difference in the amount of sleep you get. While it's unlikely to harm your baby, be aware that you may be faced with a constipated baby . . . who won't want to sleep at night.

on their sleep latency, or the time that it takes them to get to sleep. Proteins are made up of building blocks called amino acids, and the relative amount of one amino acid in particular called *tryptophan* seems to affect how babies get to sleep. Tryptophan is a precursor to a brain chemical called serotonin, which is key in determining sleep-wake cycles. Different formulas vary in the relative amount of tryptophan they contain, and this could explain differences in a baby's sleep pattern while on different formulas. Compared to breast-fed babies, formula-fed babies have relatively low amounts of tryptophan in their blood, which may explain why they tend to fall asleep more slowly.

While the solution to your baby's sleep issues may seem to be nutritional, a number of other factors are probably much more important, such as individual temperament, the environment, or whether she's had a good burp. Remember

---

Sleep and the Allergic Baby

Could a milk protein allergy be keeping your baby up at night? Perhaps. Research has shown that babies with milk protein allergy have more disruptive sleeping patterns than those without. While this may be a simple matter of poor sleep due to cramping, it's possible that immune effects on a baby's brain affect their quality of sleep. But don't count on a hypoallergenic formula to be the key to a full night's sleep. Babies get restless at night for a number of reasons, and allergy usually has other symptoms that are more obvious, such as rash, congestion, or blood in the stool.

that supplements or sleep aids containing tryptophan should never be used in babies. If your child won't sleep, talk to your doctor, since the problem is unlikely to be an amino acid issue.

BINKIES, BOTTLES, AND NIPPLES

There are so many bottle systems on the market. How do I choose?

Considering that the number of bottle systems on the market is surpassed only by the number of infant formulas, it's easy to see how the new parent can become confused. Less air, no air, smaller bubbles, easier flow—the claims made by each manufacturer are tempting, especially for the parent of a colicky baby. So really what's the difference? They're not significant. But before we jump to conclusions, let's look at the bottles and nipples separately.

A baby's bottle has one job and one job only: to store milk until inverted. Once inverted, the milk is delivered to the nipple and the bottle's role is over. While there are different sizes, shapes, materials, and vacuum types, they should make very little difference in how the normal baby feeds. What's more important is what you like and what feels comfortable in your hand.

The nipple is an entirely different story. The nipple determines the *volume* of milk delivered to the child's mouth, the *rate* of flow, and the ease at which it comes out with each suck.

What are the Important Variables in a Nipple?
- How big is the hole?
- How soft is the nipple itself?
- How much suction needs to be applied before delivering milk?

These three components of a nipple will determine the amount of milk delivered to the back of a baby's mouth. If the hole is too small or the nipple too soft, the baby may be-

---

Fact or Fiction: The Use of Plastic Bottles Is Potentially Harmful to Babies and Should Be Avoided

Fiction. Despite concerns that bottles made of polycarbonate potentially could release plastic by products when heated, the weight of scientific evidence supports their safety. In May of 1999 the Food and Drug Administration released a statement reaffirming the safety of polycarbonate bottles despite the contrary claims of critics.

---

come frustrated and suck harder, resulting in collapse of the nipple and the inevitable swallowing of air around the inadequate nipple. Similarly, if the nipple is too firm, the baby may not be able to generate enough suction to squeeze the nipple and get the milk. This too is likely to result in squeaking and air swallowing. If the hole is too big, too much milk will be delivered to the child, resulting in choking, sputtering, and dribbling.

So how are you supposed to decide which nipple is best for your baby? This discussion isn't intended to prepare you to assess flow rates and nipple tension but rather to make you aware that nipples vary tremendously. Start with a standard nipple and don't be afraid to experiment if your baby doesn't appear to be feeding efficiently. Even the same nipple design can vary from manufacturer to manufacturer. You may notice tremendous differences in the way your child feeds based on the nipple you choose for her. Consider investing in two or three different types to see what works best.

Do bottles and nipples need to be sterilized?

Cleaning bottles and nipples in a standard dishwasher is typically adequate. Sterilization is not necessary. No matter how you clean your bottle system, remember to rinse bottles and nipples shortly after their use. The sweet residue of milk at room temperature creates a terrific breeding ground for bacteria.

Is it OK to cut the hole of a nipple to make it larger?

You shouldn't need to do this. If your child is having a difficult time sucking or is taking a long time to feed, she should be evaluated by your pediatrician or an infant feeding specialist.

What about for rice cereal? Parents often cut larger nipple holes in order allow a child to suck formula thickened with rice cereal. While this isn't a problem in most cases, be aware that changing a nipple's characteristics does change the way it delivers milk to your baby. A hole that's too large can lead to choking and vomiting. A hole that's not large enough to allow the thickened formula to pass through can lead to hard sucking, frustration, air swallowing, and gas. Remember that your best efforts to soothe baby through thickened formula may lead to different problems.

I've heard that it's not a good idea to let your child hold his bottle since it may be difficult for him to let it go when it comes time to use a cup. Is this true?
Some pediatricians feel that the attachment that comes with allowing a baby to hold her own bottle can lead to difficulty when weaning to a cup. While it's true that infants may develop a feeling of ownership over their bottle when allowed to control it, this shouldn't present a problem when it comes to transitioning to a tippy cup. The ultimate decision to transition from bottle to tippy cup (which can normally occur anytime from seven to eighteen months) is yours, and the behavioral consequences aren't significant enough to keep your baby from ever holding her own bottle.

Pacifier Rules

- Only use it when you're sure he's not hungry
- Never tie it around his neck
- Never make your own pacifier
- Only use pacifiers of one-piece design
- Never use honey on a pacifier
- Use the proper size pacifier—most pacifiers come in two sizes
- Remember that a pacifier is for the baby's benefit, not yours

---

Are pacifiers bad for babies?
No, pacifiers are not bad for babies. While some would like to associate the use of pacifiers with a future of debilitating dependency and insecurity, nothing could be further from the truth. Ap-

propriate use of a pacifier will not lead to any unusual emotional attachment.

Pacifiers do have the potential to affect speech development when used beyond the second year of life. During this time children often try to speak around them instead of removing them to articulate properly.

Is it true that pacifiers can lead to crooked teeth and an abnormal bite?

How pacifiers affect dental development depends on the frequency and intensity of their use. Most children who use pacifiers regularly even into their third year will rarely go on to require orthodontic work. And despite the availability of orthodontic pacifiers, there is little you will be able to do to influence your child's future dentition besides limiting pacifier use to the first two years of life.

When should a baby stop using a pacifier?

Most babies will give up their pacifiers on their own between the ages of seventeen and twenty-two months. Socializing with other children his or her age often will encourage more age-appropriate behavior (unless, of course, your child socializes with a group of pacifier-dependent three-year-olds). Consider restricting pacifier use to nap time when your baby may need the most comfort.

In general, the earlier you decide to help your child to become independent from her pacifier, the easier it is. Keep in mind that, for a toddler, a pacifier is a terrible thing to lose.

Fact or Fiction: Pacifiers Cause Ear Infections

Possibly. While *cause* may be a bit strong, there certainly appears to be a connection. One recent study showed a 30 percent higher incidence of ear infections in children who use pacifiers. This finding may be due to pressure changes that occur between the middle ear and the mouth. If ear infections tend to be a problem for your child, you may want to consider restricting pacifier use to bed- and nap-time.

Try to replace it with some other object of comfort, such as a special blanket or stuffed toy. If all else fails, the best option is to simply misplace the pacifier. While this may precipitate two to three days of binky withdrawal, it should be the end of it.

WATER

I occasionally give my baby a bottle of water because I'm concerned he may not be getting enough fluid. Is this necessary?

While giving your child an occasional bottle of water is unlikely to do him harm, it's probably unnecessary. During the first six months, your baby gets enough fluid from breast milk or infant formula. Healthy infants usually require no supplemental water except when exposed to unusually hot weather. Even in this situation, water should be limited to approximately four ounces per day in children under six months. Once a child reaches six months and is eating a reasonable amount of solids, his need for fluid other than breast milk or formula will increase. Given the concentration of nutrients in some baby foods, additional fluid is necessary to maintain a healthy balance of minerals in the blood. Between six and twelve months, a baby's supplemental fluid intake probably should be limited to ten to twelve ounces a day.

Is it necessary that a baby's water (or the water used to prepare his formula) contain fluoride?

No. Fluoride supplementation isn't recommended for bottle- or breast-fed babies under the age of six months.

Does water need to be boiled before it's given to a baby?

Most authorities would agree that the water used to prepare infant formula should be boiled for the infant less than three months of age. Outbreaks of infectious diarrhea related to contaminated municipal water supplies are reported occasionally in the United States, but the risk is minimal and doesn't warrant aggressive sterilization for the older infant and child.

How to Sterilize Water

To sterilize water properly, bring it to a boil for a full two minutes. Don't boil for any longer since the minerals and impurities naturally found in the water can become concentrated to levels dangerous for baby.

And while you may think that baby is safe with bottled water, keep in mind that there are no standards regulating its quality or purity. If you're convinced that your bottled water actually came from two miles beneath the Swiss Alps, then you're probably OK. Otherwise, tap water is likely just as good.

GROWING BABIES

How much weight should a baby gain per day?

During the first four months of life, you can expect your baby to gain about an ounce a day or approximately one and a half to two pounds per month. Her birth weight should double by four months. Her length should increase by one to one and a half inches per month. These are estimates, of course. Your child's growth should be monitored by your physician on a growth chart. This allows a better view of what's happening and allows the doctor to compare her growth with that of other children her age.

Growth Points

- At birth the average baby boy is 20 inches long, has a head circumference of 13¾ inches, and weighs 7½ pounds. The average girl is a half pound smaller.
- Babies gain about 1 ounce a day during the first three months of life.
- Most babies double their birth weight by four months and triple their birth weight by their first birthday.
- Babies grow about 10 inches during their first year and another 4 to 5 inches during their second year.

Do big babies make big adults?

Generally speaking, a baby's height and weight have little to do with how she'll actually grow. During the first several months an infant's size is more likely to be determined by prenatal factors such as maternal nutrition, the size of the uterus, and length of gestation. During the first two years, children often will correct their weight and length to meet what their genetic potential has in store for them. By two, most toddlers will settle into a growth pattern that will stay with them until puberty. From there, a child's growth spurt during puberty and ultimate body type will be dictated by how big Mom and Dad are.

During my baby's two-week checkup she was only slightly heavier than her birth weight. Is this normal?

This is entirely normal. Babies typically lose weight during the first several days of life due to the loss of extra body water accumulated during gestation. After the loss of this extra fluid, babies begin packing on the pounds as they should. Formula-fed infants come back to their birth weight at about ten days while breast-fed infants come back to baseline closer to two weeks.

Do breast-fed infants grow differently from bottle-fed infants?

During the first three months of life, breast-fed infants tend to be chunkier than their bottle-fed counterparts. After three months and on through the end of the first year, breast-fed infants tend to be slightly leaner, or thinner, than bottle-fed infants. To the average observer, however, these differences are difficult to discern. These subtle differences that nutritional specialists have observed should have no role in deciding whether to breast- or bottle-feed.

My pediatrician told me that my baby was "in the twenty-fifth percentile for height and weight." What does this mean?

Your pediatrician got this figure from a standard pediatric growth curve, which should be part of her medical record. Growth curves provide a way for us to compare a child's height and weight with all other children her age. Being "in the twenty-fifth percentile" means that if you were to make this comparison, she would be smaller than 75 percent of them and bigger than 25 percent of them. Some parents wrongly believe that being less than average is somehow a problem. Keep in mind that someone has to be in the twenty-fifth percentile. And think how boring it would be if everybody were the same size.

Which percentile a child falls in is less important than a child's overall growth pattern, which can be determined only by following a child's weight over a period of time. Children generally tend to follow along one part of the growth curve, meaning that their growth velocity is normal. Deviation from, say, the seventy-fifth percentile to the twenty-fifth percentile over the course of a few months may indicate that the child's growth velocity is decreasing. This usually warrants some investigation.

EATING EARLY: FEEDING THE PREMATURE INFANT

My son was recently born premature at thirty-three weeks. How soon will I be able to feed him like a normal baby?
This question reflects the wishes of all parents of prematures: When will my child do the things that normal babies do? This is most evident when it comes to providing a baby with one of her most basic needs—food. While we'd like to encourage our preemie babies to feed like big, chubby term babies, unfortunately they have their own agenda, which is dictated by what their little brains and bodies allow. Most prematures lack the strength and mouth coordination to suck with efficiency from a breast or bottle until they're at about thirty-three to thirty-four weeks gestation or three and a half pounds. This, of course, varies significantly from baby to baby and is affected by other problems the baby may have, such as lung disease. Ask your neonatologists—they should be able to predict when oral feeding may begin based on how your baby is doing and what sort of premature prob-

lems she may be struggling with. Preemies often give clues that they are ready to try oral feedings. They may begin to wake up around feeding time, root, or seem more interested in the pacifier.

What does it mean to *gavage feed* a baby?

When premature babies begin feeding from the breast or bottle, they often lack the strength, endurance, and coordination to take in enough milk to meet their needs for growth. Consequently they need a little help. This is done with the help of a feeding tube, which provides babies that which they can't take on their own. This is referred to as gavage feeding. Since most young preemies are dependent on their noses for breathing, feeding tubes are often placed through the mouth (orogastric tubes). Babies closer to term are able to tolerate the placement of a tube into the nose and down into the stomach (nasogastric tube). These can be kept in place with tape for days at a time before needing replacement.

How important are pacifiers to the premature baby?

While many parents have a tendency to look on the pacifier as something to perhaps be avoided, it may have a role in the care of the premature. Studies have shown that the soothing effect of pacifiers may improve pain control, blood oxygenation, and blood pressure during times of stress. It also has been suggested that pacifiers smooth the preemie's transition to oral feeds and improve weight gain. Whether supported by studies or not, babies have the natural capacity to suck their thumbs beginning at around five months' gestation, and it seems natural to allow them the pleasure and the potential benefits that a pacifier may bring.

Our baby was fed entirely by vein for the first few weeks after she was born. Does this nutrient mixture provide everything a baby needs, or does it just hold them over until they can be fed like normal babies?

Babies under the age of about twenty-eight weeks lack the ability to fully tolerate food in the intestines. It's around this time that babies begin to develop *migrating motor complexes*, or the waves of squeezing that push milk through the intestinal tract. Because of their intestinal immaturity, babies under the age of approximately twenty-eight weeks are fed by vein with what's referred to as total parenteral nutrition (TPN). TPN provides babies with all of their nutritional needs until such a time that they are well enough and mature enough to be fed with milk. Babies placed on properly prepared TPN need no other nutritional supplementation to grow and develop.

Our premature baby has been maintained on total parenteral nutrition for the past two weeks. Things have gone fine but we get the sense from the nurses and neonatologists that there's some urgency to get her off of it. Is it dangerous?

As wonderful as it may seem, TPN does have a number of drawbacks in preemies. Among those is the catheters used to deliver TPN. Parenteral nutrition put into a catheter that slips into the wrong position can cause damage to organs, such as the liver. The venous access that babies maintain through their umbilical cords is also a prime site for infection. As long as a baby needs TPN, she needs vein access. So the sooner we can get babies off of parenteral nutrition and onto more natural forms of feeding, the better off they are.

TPN's delicate balance of sugar, protein, minerals, and vitamins presents its own risks. Its use in extremely premature infants requires a great deal of experience and monitoring to avoid the serious metabolic derangements that can occur when mixed improperly. And as with any compound or medication prepared and delivered by humans, TPN solutions can be the subject of human error. Fortunately, most neonatal intensive care nurseries have TPN teams consisting of dieticians, pharmacists, and physicians whose sole responsibility is the proper preparation and monitoring of TPN.

Finally, when used for more than a few weeks (as in babies who are very sick or have had extensive surgery), babies are at risk for impaired bile flow in the liver, referred to as *TPN cholestasis*. Babies with TPN cholestasis appear slightly jaundiced at first but it tends to intensify the longer the baby remains on TPN. In time, this accumulation of bile in the liver leads to liver cell injury. Most babies will recover from mild liver injury so long as they're off their TPN within two to three months after it's started. It's not known exactly why babies develop this problem, although it does appear to improve with the start of feeds. Even small amounts of feeding through a tube helps prevent this common complication of TPN use.

Is breast milk an appropriate source of nutrition for premature babies?

Breast milk is the preferred source of nutrition for newborns regardless of their age. This is especially true of premature infants. The presence of active enzymes in breast milk enhances digestion and helps with maturation of the growing intestine. The fat found in human milk is absorbed easier than that found in formulas. And just like any breast-fed baby, preemies benefit from the infection-fighting qualities and development-enhancing features that human milk offers.

Despite the breast-milk-is-the-perfect-food pitch, preemies do need a little help. When considering breast milk as a source of nutrition for the premature infant, it's important to keep in mind that a preemie's nutritional needs are very different from that of a full-term baby. And while the milk of a mother miraculously adapts to the needs of her premature baby with higher protein and other essential minerals, some help is still needed to insure proper growth. To address this issue, it's recommended that babies younger than thirty-five weeks' gestation and those smaller than 1,500 grams receive breast milk supplemented with fortifier. While the decision regarding your preemie's complex nutritional needs is ultimately that of your neonatologist, be sure to make your feelings known.

How does premature infant formula differ from regular infant formula?

Preemies have digestive systems that require special care, and the formulas used to feed them address those special needs. Here's what makes them different:

- *Protein.* Premature infants have a greater need for protein than full-term infants and consequently their formulas contain more. The protein used is modified cow's milk protein.
- *Fat.* The fat blends of preterm formulas are designed to compensate for the fact that preemies lack the ability to digest and absorb fats in the same way full-term infants do. Up to half the fat used in these formulas consists of a special type of fat called medium chain triglycerides (MCT), which doesn't require much for babies of any age to absorb.
- *Minerals and vitamins.* Most of a fetus's calcium, phosphorus, and magnesium is accumulated during the final trimester of pregnancy, and preemies are cheated of these due to their early delivery. Preterm formulas account for this by additional supplementation of these minerals. Sodium is another mineral that preemies need more of due to the immaturity of their kidneys. They lose more sodium than the average baby and in turn need more of it in their formula.
- *Calories.* Since premature babies need more calories than full-term babies, their formula has to be a little more potent. Consequently most preemie formulas contain approximately 20 percent more calories than standard infant formulas. Calorie-rich formula is also helpful since the volume that their tiny stomachs take is limited.

How long does a premature baby need a preterm formula?

Babies need the specially tuned features of preterm formula as long as they're preemies . . . and sometimes a bit longer. While we would like to think that a baby's nutritional shortcomings stay behind in the nursery when they go home, they still have catching up to do after they reach their due date. The effects of prematurity on a baby's mineral stores as well as their need for calories has led to the popularity of what are referred to as *transitional formulas*. As the name suggests, these formulas provide infants with a source of nutrition somewhere between premature formula and full-term infant formula. They're recommended for use once a preemie is close to her due date and doesn't require the special formulation that premature formula offers. Most babies are able to switch from a transitional formula to standard infant formula once they are one to two months beyond their due date.

SPITS, URPS, AND WET BURPS

What is gastroesophageal reflux?
Reflux describes a condition where the contents of the stomach come back up the swallowing tube where it doesn't belong. The result is a wet burp or spitup.

How common is it?
Nearly every baby spits up from time to time because *nearly all babies have reflux*. If you don't believe this, then pay a visit to your local nursery and see how many of the nurses are brave enough to burp a newborn without an absorbent cloth on her shoulder. And even if a baby doesn't spit up, it's very likely there's reflux there that you can't see. While the majority of babies spit up without difficulty, a small number will develop feeding, growth, or respiratory problems from their reflux.

Why is reflux so common in babies?
There are a number of reasons why reflux is so common:

- *Immature motility*. Just as a baby's arms and legs are uncoordinated, so is the emptying of the stomach. Sometimes it takes weeks for the normal squeezing pattern of the stomach to get in rhythm. Until that normal pattern of intestinal squeezing gets going, milk can sit in the stomach longer than normal and has a greater chance to come back up where it doesn't belong.

- *Baby's posture.* Babies spend most of their time horizontal, making it easier to reflux.
- *Liquid diet.* Lie on your back all day, take an all-liquid diet, and see if you don't feel like spitting up.
- *Air swallowing.* Babies naturally have poor coordination when it comes to sucking and swallowing. This leads to swallowing air and gas bubbles in the stomach. This distention and bloating leads to heartburn.

How do I know if my baby has reflux?

Since nearly all babies have reflux to some degree, the more important question is: How do I know if my baby has *significant* reflux? The following symptoms may indicate that your tot has more than a simple case of the spits:

- *Difficulty feeding.* Reflux can cause burning and irritation of the esophagus (swallowing tube), which causes babies to feed poorly and act irritable. Babies with this form of baby heartburn often will arch and pull off the nipple shortly after starting a feed.
- *Irritability.* The irritability of reflux is worse after feeds and is usually characterized by arching and head turning. You may notice frowns or grimacing with swallowing or after a burp.
- *Frequent hiccups.* While all babies will have hiccups from time to time, babies with reflux tend to have them often. These are caused by bloating of the stomach from swallowed air and spasm of the esophagus from the irritation of the refluxed stomach acid.
- *Congestion and breathing problems.* Chronic acid reflux can cause irritation of the upper airway, giving a baby symptoms of cough, wheezing, and congestion. Reflux-associated respiratory symptoms tend to be worse during the night when babies lie flat.

When does reflux go away?

Most cases of uncomplicated reflux disappear between four and twelve months of age. Solid food, vertical posture, and maturity of the intestines are all factors that help the spitting baby begin to keep it all together.

My three-month-old daughter was diagnosed with reflux, and our pediatrician has suggested medications. Is there anything that we can try before turning to medication?

There are a few things that can be done to minimize spitting up in babies with reflux.

- *Frequent burping*. Try to elicit a burp every one to one and a half ounces. This will prevent the accumulation of air in the stomach, which tends to predispose to reflux.
- *Positioning after feeds*. Put gravity on your side and keep your baby in a vertical position for at least twenty minutes after feeding. This means having the baby upright in a complete vertical position on your shoulder. Some parents think that having their baby in a car seat or infant carrier after feeds constitutes upright positioning. Unfortunately, the crouched position of an infant carrier has the potential to make reflux worse. That position puts the valve between the stomach and swallowing tube in the most dependent position, allowing milk to collect right where it doesn't belong.
- *Avoid rough handling during and after feeds*. Babies with reflux are more likely to spit up during the hour after feeds.
- *Elevate the head of the crib*. Elevating the head of a baby's crib puts gravity on your side by helping keep stomach contents down where they belong. Unfortunately, this works only for the first few weeks of life. After two months or so babies begin to move in their cribs, meaning that their heads can potentially wind up on the down side of the crib, thereby defeating the purpose.
- *Put her to sleep on her side*. Many babies with reflux will do better sleeping on their right side than on their back, a

position that may help facilitate emptying of the stomach. (The stomach empties to the right side.) This sort of propping works only for the first several weeks of life. After that time babies move about on their own and could wind up on their tummies.

While these simple measures tend to make things better, they are unlikely to make your child's reflux disappear completely. If your child exhibits any of the signs of chronic reflux, such as nighttime cough, chronic congestion, difficulty feeding, irritability, or poor weight gain, she may need to be treated with reflux medications.

My neighbor is a retired pediatrician and he says that reflux wasn't nearly as common twenty years ago as it is today. Why is this? Is it something in the environment or perhaps the way we're feeding babies?

Described by some as a hidden epidemic, reflux certainly has taken hold in recent years as a common diagnosis for babies. The question is: Is there actually more reflux these days, or are we identifying it more readily? My guess is that it's the latter, although there are no good studies looking at reflux then and now to prove what's really going on. When you talk to the old-time pediatricians and describe a fussy-feeding baby with frequent spitting, he or she would most likely describe that as a normal condition of infancy—and for good reason. Reflux truly is a normal condition of infancy and comes under the disease category only when a baby can't feed, grow, or breathe properly.

As our tricks and tools for diagnosing and treating the subtle variants of reflux have improved, so has our interest in looking for it. Parents read and hear about it and want to know if their child has it. Pediatricians sometimes enjoy the satisfaction of labeling a condition for tired, concerned parents who want answers. Pediatric gastroenterology has evolved so that we have small endoscopes for investigating the complications of reflux and pH meters for diagnosing the trickiest cases. The nutrition and pharmaceutical industry has gotten into the mix with new formulas and wonder drugs. We've created a cottage industry of sorts that seems to perpetuate itself. Whether it's right or wrong, we should be reassured that reflux is less likely a consequence of global warming and nothing more than a new way of looking at an old problem.

Does rice cereal prevent reflux?

A number of home-style recommendations for calming fussiness have been passed along for generations. The most common of these is the addition of rice cereal to formula in order to minimize gastroesophageal reflux. And despite the fact that this practice seems to be promoted primarily by grandmothers, pediatricians have been known to advise the use of rice cereal for spitting up in infants as early as a month after birth.

While it makes sense that thick formula should stay put, the addition of rice cereal to a baby's bottle does little to prevent acid reflux. This fact has been proven with well-controlled clinical studies comparing babies with and without rice cereal in their formula. It has been noted, however, that while spitting up may be no different when rice cereal is added, those babies tend to cry less, and there's something to be said for that.

Thickening of Formula Can Lead to Overfeeding

Keep in mind that while we tend to think of formula thickening as a generally benign intervention, it does add calories that a baby doesn't necessarily need. And considering that it's unlikely to make a significant impact on sleeping or spitting, be careful with how much you add. Your baby shouldn't need more than 2 teaspoons of cereal per ounce of formula. This alone will add an extra 10 calories per ounce to formula that's already 20 calories per ounce. That's a 50 percent increase in calories!

I've heard that chronic reflux can injure a baby's swallowing tube. How do I know if this is happening in my baby?

Parents frequently are worried about the long-term effect of stomach acid exposure on a baby's esophagus. This isn't an issue in the majority of infants with reflux because the reflux typically isn't severe enough, and most children outgrow it before developing any serious irritation to the esophagus. Children who are sick from their reflux (weight loss, feeding problems, chronic lung problems) or those who continue to spit beyond the first year should be evaluated for esophagitis (inflammation of the esophagus).

Knowing whether a child's symptoms represent serious esophagitis or just plain bad reflux is impossible based on history alone. It's usually necessary to look directly at the child's esophagus with a special instrument called an endoscope. This is done by a pediatric gastroenterologist in an outpatient setting.

My six-week-old seems to have the hiccups constantly. They seem worse after eating, and I'm concerned that they're making her uncomfortable. What's causing this and is there anything I can do about it?

Hiccups represent spasm or twitching of the diaphragm (the large muscle that separates the chest from the abdomen). The diaphragm normally contracts regularly to allow us to take in even, slow breaths. When the diaphragm contracts or twitches suddenly, a small amount of air is taken in. As this occurs, the vocal cords immediately snap shut, causing the sound that we typically associate with a hiccup. This closing of the vocal cords probably represents an effort by the body to prevent the inhalation of food during the hiccup.

Despite the fact that all babies experience hiccups from time to time, it's not clear why hiccups occur. We do know that they tend to occur more often during and after feeding. We tend to see hiccups more frequently in children with reflux. While remedies abound, there's little else besides patience and perhaps frequent burping that have been found to help the infant with hiccups.

When my daughter spits up, it comes out her nose. Is this cause for concern?

While regurgitated stomach contents coming from the nose may seem particularly dramatic, it really has no relevance to the severity of a baby's reflux. It probably relates more to a normal variation in the child's anatomy than anything else.

What does it mean when my child throws up curdled milk?

The regurgitation of curdled milk is often considered an ominous sign by new parents but is entirely normal. When milk protein is exposed to the acidic environment of the stomach, it congeals or curdles to form cheesy lumps. If you had the opportunity to examine the inside of a normal baby's stomach after eating, you would find that milk normally forms these small lumps as part of digestion.

My six-month-old has reflux and has been treated with medications since three months without success. I've heard that an operation sometimes is used when babies don't get well. How do I know if my child needs this?

Once the decision has been made that a baby's reflux is bad enough to warrant treatment, the first step is to begin a trial of medications. In most cases this consists of two types of medications: an antacid to decrease the burning sensation a baby experiences and a medication to help the stomach squeeze and empty. Generally this combination leads to some improvement in the baby's symptoms within a week or two. This improvement usually makes the symptoms tolerable enough until the reflux improves on its own. Sometimes, however, medications have very little impact on an infant's reflux and we're then faced with a very important question: How much further are we going to go to fix this problem?

The answer to this question depends on what kind of problems the baby has experienced. The complications of reflux that get pediatricians and gastroenterologists excited include severe choking, chronic lung disease, apnea (occasional stopping of breathing), inability to feed, and poor growth. Once a baby has demonstrated one or any combination of these symptoms and treatment has failed with medications at the appropriate doses, then consideration is given to other treatments, such as surgery.

The operation to fix reflux is referred to as a *fundoplication*. This is an operation performed by a pediatric surgeon in which the top of the stomach is wrapped or pinched around the bottom of the esophagus (swallowing tube). This tightens the area between the bottom of the swallowing tube and the top of the stomach and prevents any further reflux. The degree of wrap that a surgeon does depends on a number of factors, including the degree of reflux the child is experiencing, her long-term outlook, and any other associated problems she may have.

My pediatrician told me my son has reflux, but he has never spit up. How can this be?
Your pediatrician isn't a quack (at least on the basis of this issue). The world is full of children with reflux who have never spit up. Spitting up or regurgitation is only one of a number of symptoms that lead pediatricians to think of reflux as a problem in babies. Sometimes reflux can show itself as nothing more than a feeding problem that causes babies to pull from the nipple and struggle with the bottle. Other times reflux can lead to wheezing and chronic cough with nothing else to suggest an intestinal problem. Reflux can imitate a number of other conditions in babies, and it's your pediatrician's job to try to figure what those problems are.

A Formula with Added Rice: When and Why?

Just when you thought it was safe to go back to the formula aisle, one manufacturer has come up with a thickened formula intended to help the spitting baby. "AR formula" comes premixed with rice starch in order to provide a thicker, more-difficult-to-spit milk for babies. At ten times the thickness and at about the cost of regular formula, it's likely to do little else than save you from adding those pesky rice flakes to your baby's bottle. Despite a limited number of studies suggesting success, there's no solid evidence that the addition of rice to a baby's formula does anything to improve reflux.

Considering that AR formula represents a nutritionally complete alternative for infants with reflux, it may be worth a shot. Like so many things with kids, it can't hurt and might help.

Is there one type of formula proven to help babies with reflux?

Despite the desperate efforts of the formula industry, there isn't any one formula clearly proven to be of benefit for reflux. The only form of infant nutrition known to be advantageous to babies with reflux is breast milk. When formula-feeding parents hear this, they often feel immense guilt over the fact that they may have caused their child's reflux through choosing to formula-feed. While it's true that your baby may have had milder reflux on breast milk, formula-feeding didn't cause the reflux. It likely would have been there no matter how you chose to feed.

Chapter 2

Figuring Out Formulas

When it comes to the everyday issues facing the new parent, everyone wonders if they're doing the right thing. If you're one of them, you're not alone. But what happens when a mother can't get her questions answered about her baby's colicky behavior or potential allergy? Maybe she feels that her questions and concerns are foolish. Perhaps the relationship with her pediatrician is not as open as she would like or she doesn't feel confident of the answers she gets. In this setting parents often take matters into their own hands. And in the case of the formula-fed child, that often means making a formula change. For some babies, one change is enough. For others, formula and its potential for changing a baby's disposition leads to formula roulette.

What drives a parent's decision to play musical formulas and change to that latest and greatest new milk? Usually it's desperation and the lack of any other variable in a baby's life for tweaking. Babies don't (appear to) do much else other than eat, sleep, and fill their diapers. We can't control their sleep; it's tough to regulate their bowel movements; but feeding, ah yes, the feeding is in our control. So when things get out of hand and baby's making *us* gassy, fussy, cranky, and fidgety, we change their formula.

Unfortunately, most things that make babies cranky are unrelated to their formula. Ultimately, the problems that cause a baby to be profoundly fussy resolve, and if you change formulas frequently enough, you're likely to time the resolution of the baby's problem with the start of one of the formulas. Go ahead and make your formula changes, but read on and be informed about what you're doing. Most important, understand that all that glitters isn't gold . . . or a better formula.

FORMULA BASICS

What's the difference among all of the formulas that I see displayed in the grocery store?

Considering the variety of formulas available, it's easy to become confused when choosing one for your baby. And that's one good reason why all decisions concerning formula should be made only after speaking with your pediatrician. Keep in mind that despite the number of different brands available, most formulas fall into one of three basic categories: cow's-milk-based, soy, and specialized.

Cow's-Milk-Based Formula

This is the most basic type of infant formula and the standard formula that infants are offered if you choose not to breast-feed. It accounts for approximately 80 percent of formula sold. Although it's based on cow's milk, it's manufactured in such a way to be safe for a baby's digestive system. The milk is hydrolyzed (partially predigested) to be less irritating, and the normal milk fat is replaced with vegetable oils, which are more easily digested. Extra lactose is added to make the amount of sugar similar to that in breast milk.

Soy Formula

Soy formula differs from standard formula in that it's manufactured with a different protein (soy) and different sugar (sucrose or modified starch). This formula is used during episodes of acute diarrhea, when some babies are temporarily intolerant to the regular milk sugar, lactose. And if you're a strict vegetarian who isn't breast-feeding, this may be the formula for you since it contains no animal products. Soy formula represents a sound nutritional alternative to breast milk and standard formula, although it tends to be more expensive.

Formula Forms: Ready-to-Feed, Concentrate, and Powder

Most infant formulas are available in one of three forms: ready-to-feed, concentrate, and powder. Ready-to-feed preparations are the most convenient and also the most expensive. The concentrate form is less expensive and typically is made by mixing 1:1 with water. If you use concentrate, be sure to add the proper amount of water. Adding too much water can dilute the nutrition available from formula while adding too little can dangerously concentrate protein and certain minerals, putting a baby's kidneys at risk for damage.

The powdered form is the least expensive and requires mixing with the proper amount of water until completely dissolved. The advantage of this form, besides the cost, is that it's lightweight and good for toting. You can put the proper amount of powder in a bottle, get on your way, and mix it with water right before use.

Many parents use powder formula when their infants are younger and taking smaller amounts per feeding only to switch to liquid concentrate when older. This may be more convenient when infants want their feeding now, cold, instead of later, warm.

Specialized Formulas

There are a number of formulas available for infants who have unusual conditions (severe allergy or digestive problems). Some such formulas contain a predigested form of milk protein that is much less irritating to babies with milk allergy. Others contain a special form of fat that's more easily absorbed by children who have diseases of the pancreas or liver. Specialized formulas are reserved for babies with serious problems and should be used only under the careful supervision of your pediatrician.

Our grocery store carries its own line of infant formula, and it's considerably less expensive than the brand-name formulas. We're probably best off staying away from these generic formulas, right?

Wrong. Most store-brand formulas are manufactured by Wyeth Nutritionals, a respected formula manufacturer that has been around for years and only recently chose to sell its formula under the label of major stores and chains. While a store brand may seem like second best, the Food and Drug Administration regulates the manufacture of all infant formulas to ensure that they meet standards of composition and quality. Consequently, store-brand standard and soy formulas are as nutritionally complete as any formula available. The money that store-brand formulas save in marketing and promotion is passed on to the consumer, which could cut your formula bill by 40 percent during your first year.

My pediatrician referred to my child's formula as a "cow's-milk-based formula." How does this differ from milk out of the carton?
Parents are often confused by the fact that we don't allow babies to have cow's milk until a year of age, yet standard infant formulas are referred to as "cow's-milk-based formulas." The terminology arises from the fact that regular infant formulas are manufactured using cow's milk protein, the same protein found in whole milk. The difference is that, before it is used, it is heated slightly and partially digested, making it less irritating to a baby's digestive system. Not only is the protein slightly predigested, the amount of protein found in infant formula is also adjusted to make it more appropriate for babies.

Infant formulas also differ from whole milk in the type of fat used. During manufacturing, the butterfat of whole milk is replaced with vegetable oils, which are more easily digested and absorbed by babies. The composition and balance of oils used in most formulas mimic the fat composition in breast milk. Fat composition in infant formulas is the subject of intense research, since it is felt that different fats and their proportions in a baby's diet may impact such things as brain and eye development.

Finally, since whole milk is high in sodium and potassium and low in iron and vitamin C, infant formulas are adjusted to contain a more appropriate balance of vitamins and minerals for the growing baby.

I have heard that if a baby takes a little from a bottle and doesn't finish the rest, it needs to be discarded. Is this true?
Yes. Bacteria from the mouth naturally contaminate the contents of the bottle during feeding. Left on their own, these

bacteria grow and multiply in the warm, sweet environment of infant formula. If you're interrupted during a feed and have to leave a bottle, it's OK to use it at room temperature for up to one hour. If there's any question, dispose of it.

Are baby formulas Kosher?

It depends on the brand of formula and your degree of observance. Most formulas produced by major manufacturers bear the Orthodox Union symbol indicating widely accepted Kashruth supervision. Most major formulas manufactured in the United States are certified Kosher-dairy with few exceptions. Certification tends to vary more for the hypoallergenic formulas.

Formula Facts

- Prior to the 1900s, most non-breast-fed babies died in the first year.
- From 1930 to 1960, evaporated milk was the most common infant formula used.
- In 1967 the American Academy of Pediatrics made the first recommendations to standardize infant formula.
- Soy formula makes up 20 percent of the formula purchased in the United States.
- Eighty-five percent of parents will provide formula for their baby at some point during the first year.
- Fifty-nine percent of formula purchased in the United States is in powder form.

Is there ever any reason for formula to be watered down?

For those of us forced to make every penny count, diluting a baby's formula may seem like a way to get more bottles for our buck. Unfortunately, there's no such thing as a free lunch (or bottle). As a general rule, formula should *never* be watered down. Remember that while it may seem like a benign practice, diluted formula shortchanges a baby on her protein, calories, and nutrients. Over a matter of weeks a baby who may seem full and satisfied can become malnourished.

Despite its long-term danger, pediatricians sometimes recommend diluting a baby's formula for a day or two during a severe diarrhea illness. The dilution limits the amount of sugar that a baby receives and may decrease the number of diarrhea stools. This practice should be limited to three

---

How Many Calories Does a Baby Need?

While I'm typically against any feeding advice that involves the use of a calcula-tor, parents occasionally ask: *How many calories does my baby need to grow?* Since babies have an innate ability to adjust their intake of calories based on what they need, the best answer is *as many as she'll take.* For the sake of argu-ment we can do the math and prove that what your baby takes is (we hope) what she needs.

Infants need approximately 100 calories per kilogram per day (there are 2.2 kilograms in a pound) during the first year. As an example, a typical two-month-old baby at 5 kilograms would need 500 calories a day for normal growth and development. Considering that the average infant formula and breast milk con-tains 20 calories per ounce, her calorie needs will be met with approximately 25 ounces per day, the typical intake for a two-month-old.

---

days and should be done only under the supervision of your pediatrician.

I've heard that formula can be concentrated for babies who don't eat enough. Is this true?

Sometimes babies fail to take in enough calories to meet their needs for growth. This can occur for any number of reasons, including feeding difficulties, chronic reflux, and prematurity to name a few. To offset a child's marginal in-take, doctors sometimes recommend the use of concentrated infant formula to increase the number of calories that a baby gets in every ounce. A common step is to concentrate for-mula from its normal twenty-calorie-per-ounce concentra-tion to twenty-four calories per ounce. This gives the baby more "bang for the buck" with each ounce taken and often makes up for deficiencies in volume. Consider the following recipes for concentrated formula, should it be recommended by your physician:

Using powder: Add 3 level, unpacked scoops of powder to 5 ounces of water.
Using liquid concentrate: Add 9 ounces of water to a full can of liquid concentrate to bring the total volume to 22 ounces.

Using ready-to-feed: Add 1 scoop of powder to every 10 ounces of standard, ready-to-feed formula.

Remember:

- Make sure all utensils and containers are clean.
- Store in the refrigerator in a covered container.
- Use within forty-eight hours of preparation.
- Discard formula remaining in each bottle after each feeding.

We normally prepare our daughter's formula from powder. Recently we bought ready-to-feed formula by the same manufacturer and found it to be darker and slightly thicker. Has it gone bad?

Ready-to-feed formulas often appear thicker than their powder-mix counterparts. This appearance is a result of the sterilization process that liquid formula must undergo in order to be safe for babies. The nutrient content is equivalent, and both forms should be equally tolerated by your baby.

I've heard that juvenile diabetes is somehow related to milk intake during childhood. Is there any truth to this?

It's been suggested that cow's-milk-based infant formulas and cow's-milk consumption in childhood promote the development of juvenile diabetes (type I diabetes). By way of background, diabetes is a disease where the insulin-producing cells in the pancreas are attacked by the immune system, rendering them functionless. It falls into a category of diseases called *autoimmune disease*—or diseases where the body attacks itself for reasons unknown. The milk-diabetes theory is that the small chunks of milk protein make it into the blood early in life and stimulate the production of antibodies, the part of our immune system responsible for recognizing and initiating the attack on foreign proteins by the body later in life. It's felt that these antibodies can cross-react with the cells in our pancreas responsible for insulin production and initiate their destruction.

While there have been studies supporting the role of early milk exposure in diabetes, there are just as many studies showing no connection. Some of the research stems from studies in animals, which may be hard to apply to humans. The clinical studies in humans have been mostly *retrospective* studies (studies based on review and recollection of a child's feeding history). As with any type of research that depends on a parent's memory of how much milk was given when, the results must be held in question. What's needed is a large, well-designed study that follows children from birth through the later years of childhood so that a tight connection (should there be one) can be made.

But if there's any question, shouldn't parents just avoid

DHA—Brain Food for Babies

Formula manufacturers are forever striving to create a formula that most closely matches mother's milk. Currently they're focusing on whether to add a compound called DHA (docosahexanoic acid) to their products. DHA helps form the structure of such tissues as the retina and the brain. Although a baby receives a great deal of DHA during the last trimester of pregnancy, DHA also is delivered through breast milk. Formulas available in the United States do not contain DHA.

Is this a problem? Perhaps, say proponents of DHA. There is some evidence to suggest that babies fed DHA-supplemented formulas have improved visual and, perhaps, cognitive functioning when compared with infants fed regular formula. In some studies breast-fed babies have been found to develop slightly higher IQs, but it is not known whether this difference is due to DHA; breast milk contains many other ingredients that formulas don't have.

Although the importance of DHA in infant nutrition still is under investigation, some international organizations have recommended that DHA and arachidonic acid (a similar acid) be added to infant formulas. In fact, some formula manufacturers in other countries—such as Japan, Germany, and the Netherlands—have been influenced by the evidence in favor of DHA and now routinely supplement their infant formulas. The American Academy of Pediatrics, however, has yet to take a position on this issue, because of the lack of conclusive evidence in DHA's favor. Despite the fact that many authorities already believe that DHA is necessary for the optimal growth and development of infants, studies are ongoing, and more work has to be done. Until the final verdict is in, the simplest answer may be to breast-feed.

cow's milk and cow's-milk formula altogether? As tempting as this logic may seem, there simply isn't enough evidence to support such a policy. Rather than take the safest approach possible, we have to base what we do on what we know to be fact. If, however, you want to use this issue as a motivator to breast-feed, all the better. Otherwise, standard infant formula shouldn't provoke anxiety should you choose to use it.

HOT AND COLD

What's the problem with using a microwave oven to warm formula or breast milk?
While it's hard to think of microwave ovens as anything less than a godsend to parents, they can present a hidden danger to babies. Any liquid heated in a microwave may be subject to onion skinning, a phenomenon where layers of liquid can heat up to high temperature. What this means is that an apparently lukewarm bottle of formula may harbor dangerously hot areas. This can lead to superficial burns of the mouth and throat and cause a child to eat poorly for days.

The best policy is to plan ahead and avoid the urgency of needing to heat a bottle right away. Placing a chilled four-ounce bottle into a bowl of hot tap water will bring baby's formula up to the perfect temperature in seven to eight minutes. If you have a penchant for gadgets, there are a variety of electric bottle warmers that will do as good a job with a lot more style, pizzazz, and expense. Finally, remember that heated formula probably makes parents happier than it does babies. Despite what Grandma says, there has yet to be a baby who's suffered in the face of a chilled bottle of formula.

Once formula has been prepared, how long is it safe to keep it at room temperature? How about in the refrigerator?
Opened or prepared formula is good for up to forty-eight hours in the refrigerator. At room temperature, formula

should be used within two to four hours. While you may get away with pushing the limits of these parameters, remember that formula can begin to harbor dangerous counts of bacteria when left open too long. When in doubt, throw it out.

Can infant formula be frozen?

Infant formula should *never* be frozen. Freezing can be detrimental to the protein and nutrients critical for growth.

Is it dangerous to give a baby chilled milk?

While we have always associated warm milk with content babies, there's no rule requiring a baby's milk be given warm. Most babies will drink chilled milk as well as they will warm milk, and temperature has no impact on its digestion.

TASTE, TOUCH, AND SMELL

When will my baby be able to taste, and can she tell the difference between formulas?

Contrary to what most new parents think, babies are able to discriminate a small variety of taste sensations from the first few hours of life, and this can hold true for formulas. From the time of birth, infants appear to be able to distinguish among sweet, sour, and bitter. This remarkable ability should, however, have little impact on what you feed or how you feed it. The taste of infant formula should vary very little from manufacturer to manufacturer as long as you're comparing similar types of formula; some babies will show a preference for soy over standard formula or vice versa. Many babies will turn their noses up at hypoallergenic formulas because of their taste and odor.

While babies may have the capacity to discriminate among formulas, the differences shouldn't be significant enough to lead to refusal of one formula over another. If you feel the need to make a formula change because your baby doesn't seem to like the taste of regular formula, it's reasonable to give soy a shot. If this produces a sour face, consult your physician before playing musical formulas—there are many reasons why babies will turn their nose up at the bottle, and flavor is least often the cause.

Is it OK to sweeten my baby's formula?

If you've never had thoughts of sweetening your baby's formula, you've probably never had the opportunity to taste it. Despite its flat, bland taste, infant formula should *never* be sweetened (except under special circumstances). Your baby's palate is not refined enough to require it, and excessive sugar can lead to slow intestinal motility, diarrhea, and tooth decay. If your baby has a problem feeding, she should be evaluated by your pediatrician.

What's the problem with using honey on a baby's pacifier or nipple?

This is an old-fashioned tip that belongs in the archives of child care. Honey is taboo for babies since it can contain spores of the organism *Clostridium botulinum*. This organism can cause a condition in babies called neonatal botulism. Babies with neonatal botulism experience difficulty feeding, weakness, and occasionally compromised breathing. This condition is, fortunately, rare due to an improved awareness of honey's risk among today's generation of parents.

How is it that adults can eat honey without problem? The level of toxin released by the rare, tainted honey isn't enough to lead to problems in adults due to their size.

EXPENSIVE AND STINKY: SPECIAL FORMULAS AND THE ALLERGIC BABY

Our son is five weeks old and for the past two weeks we have begun noticing streaks of blood and mucus mixed in with his stool. He also seems to be fussy when having a bowel movement. Is this some sort of formula reaction?

What you're describing is typical of milk protein hypersensitivity, or milk allergy, in a newborn. Despite the fact that this a fairly common problem occurring in up to 5 percent of normal infants, it's always scary seeing blood in your baby's diaper. The best way to think about milk protein hypersensitivity is as a rash or reaction of the lining of the intestine to milk protein. This reaction leads to bleeding, extra mucus production, and spasm of the colon. As with any form of colonic irritation or colitis, the process of having a bowel movement can cause colicky, crampy pain. In a baby this appears as crying and pulling up of the knees with bowel movements despite soft, even diarrhealike stools.

Beyond the intestines, babies with more severe milk allergy will show other symptoms, such as rash, eczema, nasal congestion, and wheezing. These symptoms are much less common than the bleeding and fussiness more typical of babies with garden-variety milk allergy.

Milk protein allergy in babies is treated with a hypoallergenic formula such as Nutramigen® or Alimentum®. The protein in these formulas is specially treated to be less reactive to those infants with a known sensitivity. While there are exceptions, milk protein hypersensitivity in babies is limited to the first several months of life. Infants with milk allergy typically need to remain on a hypoallergenic formula for the first five to eight months of life, after which they can be transitioned back onto a standard infant formula. Most babies will grow into their toddler years able to tolerate whole milk and other dairy products without any problem.

As with most problems, things aren't always as they seem. While your son's problem appears to be a protein hypersensitivity, there are other conditions, such as bacterial infections of the intestine, that can mimic allergy. Be sure to visit with your pediatrician before making formula changes.

How are hypoallergenic formulas different from standard formulas?
So your child has been placed on a hypoallergenic formula. What is it that makes them so special? It's all about the protein. In hypoallergenic infant formulas, the protein has been modified so as not to react with a baby's intestine. (Protein

reactivity is the basic problem in the baby with milk allergy or milk protein hypersensitivity.)

Proteins are made up of large chains of amino acids, the building blocks of protein. The body recognizes and reacts to certain sequences and arrangements of those chains of amino acids, and the result is milk protein hypersensitivity or allergy. Hypoallergenic formulas are manufactured by slightly heating and breaking down the protein so that the body doesn't recognize it in its natural form. All the pieces of the protein are there, it's just been slightly disassembled so as to fool the body. Since the amount of protein is comparable to that found in standard infant formulas, children grow and develop just fine on hypoallergenic formulas.

Standard Hypoallergenic Formulas

The standard hypoallergenic formulas Nutramigen (Mead Johnson) and Alimentum (Ross) consist of moderately digested cow's milk protein and are available in most grocery stores. These formulas represent the first line treatment in infant milk allergy.

Super-Hypoallergenic Formulas

Super-hypoallergenic formulas such as Neocate® (SHS Nutritionals) contain no intact protein and consist entirely of protein links or amino acids. They are used in babies with severe milk allergy or those who continue to have bothersome symptoms on a standard hypoallergenic formula. Neocate is available only through the manufacturer and is typically shipped to your pharmacy. It should be used only under the direct supervision of your physician.

Toddler Hypoallergenic Formulas

For the unusual infant who breaks into his second year with a persistent sensitivity to milk protein, formulas such as Neocate One+® or Elecare® take over. These formulas contain more appropriate levels of protein and vitamins for the toddler. Since true milk protein hypersensitivity beyond the first year of life is so unusual, be sure that your pediatrician

---

A Better Whey?

As a means of trying to build a better mousetrap, Carnation manufactures Goodstart®, a formula containing 100 percent hydrolyzed whey. *Whey* is one of the two major types of protein found in cow's milk; *casein* is the other. The fact that it's hydrolyzed means that it's broken down and potentially less allergenic. While it's been said that whey hydrolysates may be more gentle for a baby or empty more quickly from the stomach, these claims probably serve a marketing agenda better than they do your baby's gassy stomach. Hydrolyzed whey represents a fine protein source for any child's formula, but its qualities are not magical. It can't hurt and might help, so feel free to give it a whirl. Just don't get caught playing musical formulas.

---

is confident of the diagnosis before committing your child to one of these top-shelf toddler formulas.

As with all things in life, everything comes with a cost. In the case of the hypoallergenic formulas, the process of hydrolyzing or breaking down the milk protein leads to milk with an unpleasant taste and an even more unpleasant price tag.

Our family has a strong history of food allergy. Should I start my baby off on a hypoallergenic formula to prevent any potential reaction?

Considering that food allergy is one of the most overrated concepts of modern civilization, one must always consider a "strong family history of food allergy" as suspect. Most often in these cases a thorough family history reveals poorly documented lactose intolerance and other vague, anecdotal difficulties that families have a hard time even describing.

Even in families where there is a strong history of true, documented food allergies, babies are almost never begun on hypoallergenic formulas. The likelihood of a baby having a genetically programmed protein allergy bad enough to warrant the preventive use of a hypoallergenic formula is very small. Babies have a way of telling us if they're sensitive to milk protein. Wait until you have something to treat before committing her to months of a smelly, expensive formula.

Colic—a Nutritional Problem?

For the uninitiated reader, colic is a poorly understood condition seen in babies from a couple of weeks to three months of age. Symptoms include difficult-to-console fussiness and gas typically worse in the evening hours. One of the key diagnostic criteria is that the irritability experienced by the involved parents often rivals that of the baby's.

Parents always want to know what they can do for their baby with colic. Considering that formula or breast milk is the only thing that babies put in their mouths at this age, they're a natural target as potential colic culprits. Unfortunately, the studies done to date show no convincing connection between infant diet and colic. It is accepted, however, that there is a small subset of babies with "colic" who are actually suffering from milk protein allergy. The few studies done show that allergy accounts for no more than 10 to 15 percent of babies reported as having this frustrating problem. So while the odds are stacked against you (or your baby), a trial of Nutramigen or Alimentum may be reasonable. But don't hold your breath, and remember, three months really isn't that long.

My two-month-old daughter was put on Nutramigen four weeks ago for streaks of blood and mucus in the stool. Her bleeding and fussiness seemed to clear up after the first couple of weeks and everything was going great. Yesterday we noticed a little bit of blood when changing her diaper. Is the formula not working? Babies with milk protein hypersensitivity will sometimes react even to hypoallergenic formulas. Even though the milk protein is broken down, sometimes the most sensitive colon can't be fooled. A small amount of bleeding here and there isn't a problem as long as your baby is happy, healthy, and gaining weight. To get rid of that occasional streak of blood would require a change to a very expensive and extremely hypoallergenic formula. It doesn't appear to be necessary in this case, although this is a decision best made by your doctor or pediatric gastroenterologist.

Our child was recently seen by a pediatric gastroenterologist and placed on Neocate for ongoing rectal bleeding and rash due to a severe milk protein allergy. It looks as if this formula is going to cost us about $600 a month, and we simply can't afford

it. Our insurance claims they won't cover it. Shouldn't our insurance company pay this?

Unfortunately, it's standard practice that insurance payers in the United States don't cover nutritional products in infants. And when you look at it from the perspective of the insurance companies, it's easy to understand why. Parents frequently get wrapped up in formula switches that are recommended by their pediatricians often for ambiguous symptoms, such as gas and fussiness. If every switch to soy or lactose-free formula were deemed a medical necessity, insurance carriers would be inundated with formula claims. The red tape from this problem alone would make all of our insurance premiums prohibitive.

In the minds of most pediatric gastroenterologists and those insurance executives with any sense of compassion, Neocate represents a different story, however. Children who require the use of specialized formulas such as this often have no other option when it comes to treatment for their allergy. And it also represents a catastrophic expense for those families that are committed to its use for the several months that it may be required. Some insurance groups have recognized this problem and taken the lead by implementing policies to cover formulas like Neocate when the indications are clear. In your case, however, it seems that your insurance carrier has no such policy. Talk to your pediatric gastroenterologist, since he very likely has petitioned insurance providers in the past and likely will be willing to send a letter detailing the unusual situation your child is in. Don't be afraid to do this yourself as well. A well-written letter to the right person will frequently do more than phone calls to the receptionist. Emphasize that Neocate is a *medicinal* formula that represents a catastrophic expense to your family.

Finally, talk to the benefits coordinator of the company you work for, preferably the highest person in the ranks. See if they'll write a letter on your behalf describing your situation. If you work for a large company, most insurance carriers are willing to make concessions when one of the company heavies goes to bat for you. Usually they would rather keep your company as a client than risk losing it all over a couple of months of formula.

Isn't lactose intolerance the same thing as allergy?

This is a common source of confusion among parents and even some pediatricians. *Lactose intolerance* is a lifelong condition commonly seen starting in school-age children and young adults. It results from the loss of lactase (the enzyme responsible for digesting milk sugar) in the wall of the intestine. Since lactose can't be digested and absorbed properly, it passes all the way into the large intestine, where it gets fermented by the bacteria present there. It typically causes gas, bloating, and diarrhea when lactose is present in the diet.

Milk allergy in infants is typically a temporary condition and involves a reaction by the body to the protein found in formula or breast milk. It is quite common and is reported to occur in up to 5 percent of infants. Symptoms include blood and mucus in the stool, cramping with bowel movements, and occasionally rash and wheezing. Children with milk allergy tolerate lactose just fine.

> ### Lactose Intolerance— Babies Just Don't Get It
>
> Everybody talks about it, parents love to label their kids with it, pediatricians promote it, and formula companies support it. Unfortunately, babies just don't get it. Babies born with lactose intolerance are exceptionally rare. In fact, when a baby is discovered without lactase, the proper enzyme for digesting the milk sugar lactose, it's an event reportable to doctors and scientists in the medical literature. While babies may temporarily become lactose intolerant after an intestinal infection, this lasts only for a week or two.

If true lactose intolerance is so rare in babies, why are there infant formulas specially designed for lactose intolerance?

This is a darned good question. Market decisions often are driven by demand and not necessarily by what is physiologically or scientifically sound. Many parents have rigid perceptions about their baby's digestive system based on family history or what they've heard from friends, neighbors, or grandmothers. Consequently, when pediatricians are faced with a cranky baby and an even crankier parent, it's sometimes easier to try something that "can't hurt, might help."

Does it mean you're a cranky mother if your pediatrician puts your baby on a lactose-free formula? Not necessarily. Some pediatricians themselves mix up the lactose intolerance and milk allergy issue. For others, the time constraints placed on them by managed care make extensive education difficult if not impossible.

My son spits frequently. Could this be a sign of milk allergy?

While spitting can indicate allergy in some cases, it's unlikely to be the case without other symptoms of allergy, such as blood and mucus in the stools, cramping with bowel movements, rash, or wheezing.

All babies have some spitting, which is usually the result of mild reflux. Reflux is not an allergy problem, and formula changes are unlikely to do anything to change the spitting.

Is there anything that can be done to improve the horrible flavor of hypoallergenic formula?

Infants and parents alike are often repulsed by the odor and flavor of hypoallergenic formulas. This unpleasant taste is a natural outcome of the protein digestion that is necessary to make the formula hypoallergenic. Despite how unappealing these formulas may be, getting the seriously allergic baby to take them can be very important.

Fortunately, most babies will take hypoallergenic formula as well as standard formula within twenty-four to forty-eight hours if given nothing else to drink. It seems that the infants closer to three months of age or older have more refined tastes and are more resistant to the flavor. I often encourage parents to wait several feedings to see if their infant will give in.

If patient persistence fails, try adding 1 drop of vanilla extract to each four-ounce bottle of formula. While most vanilla extracts have an alcohol base, the amount a baby re-

ceives in one drop isn't anything to worry about. If this
doesn't do the trick, consider adding a quarter- to a half-
packet of Nutrasweet® to each bottle. While sweeteners, natural or artificial, typically are considered taboo for babies,
the consequences of ongoing allergy make this the exception. Limited amounts of Nutrasweet in this setting are safe
for most babies, but talk to your pediatrician or gastroenterologist before trying this. Under no circumstances should
children with phenylketonuria (PKU) be given Nutrasweet,
since it contains phenylalanine, a chemical additive not allowed in individuals with PKU.

Is soy formula the formula of choice for babies with milk allergy?

Most authorities agree that soy formula is not the formula of
choice for babies with milk protein hypersensitivity. Some
studies investigating this problem have shown that up to 50
percent of infants who react to milk protein also will react to

---

The Vast Soy Conspiracy

Is there a vast soy conspiracy in America? Maybe so. Everyone loves soy formula, but the truth of the matter is that no baby really needs it. In fact, if you ask
any self-respecting pediatric nutritionist what soy formula is really used for,
you'll have a hard time getting a straight answer. While it gives all pediatricians
a warm fuzzy feeling to dispense this during a diarrhea illness, research doesn't
support that it really does anything. A genetic disorder called galactosemia warrants its use, but kids with this disease are as rare as hen's teeth. And no discussion of oddball formulas would be complete without some mention of colic.
While soy formula has been marketed as a formula for colicky babies, it has
been suggested by some that the strongest indication for the use of soy formula
is a colicky parent.

Whatever it is soy formula does to deserve such a coveted place on our grocery store shelves may remain one of the great unsolved mysteries of the modern era, right up there with the JFK assassination and Colonel Sanders's secret
recipe. If nothing else, its mysterious presence in our lives should serve as a re-
minder that what we do as parents and pediatricians sometimes makes absolutely no sense.

soy protein. So if your baby has signs of milk allergy, you're playing the odds by switching to soy. A casein hydrolysate formula such as Nutramigen or Alimentum is a better choice.

I've heard that soy formula contains small amounts of hormone. Is this true, and is it dangerous?

While most parents are unaware of it, soy formulas contain naturally occurring, plant-derived substances referred to as phytoestrogens. Phytoestrogens are naturally occurring hormonelike substances found in a variety of foods, including apples, wheat, and soy. Soybeans happen to contain the highest levels of phytoestrogens, and these levels carry through to infant formula despite the processing that occurs. While these are true hormones, they don't appear to have quite the same effect as we typically associate with hormones. They are touted to offer potential therapy for a variety of conditions, from cancer to heart disease, although little scientific evidence exists to support their widespread clinical use.

Despite concerns over their presence in infant formulas, very few studies have examined the effects of phytoestrogens in babies. It is known that infants digest and absorb phytoestrogens differently from adults due to immaturity of the digestive tract. Nonetheless, infants fed soy formula have been found to have phytoestrogen derivatives in their blood. Cow's milk and breast milk also contain phytoestrogens but not to the degree found in soy formula.

Despite their use for over three decades, there is no evidence that soy formula causes babies any problem. In fact, studies done with newborn rats have suggested that early exposure to certain phytoestrogens conferred protection against later breast cancer. It's also known that populations who consume large amounts of soy and plant-based products show a lower incidence of such hormone-dependent cancers as breast and prostate cancer.

Why do some pediatricians recommend soy formula for babies with stomach infections?

To understand why pediatricians sometimes make this decision, it's important to understand what happens to a child during an intestinal viral infection. When viruses attack the intestine during a typical gastroenteritis, they temporarily destroy its delicate lining. This lining contains special enzymes for the digestion and absorption of sugars. If the sugars that are

> **Soy Milk Isn't for Infants**
>
> *Soy milk* that can be purchased in your grocery store's dairy case should not be confused with *soy-based infant formula*. Unlike soy-based infant formula, soy milk lacks the proper balance of vitamins and nutrients needed by babies. Several cases of severe malnutrition have been reported in infants fed soy milk as their sole source of nutrition. As with cow's milk out of the carton, soy milk out of the carton is fine for babies over a year.

part of a baby's diet don't get absorbed properly, they pass into the colon and get fermented by the bacteria that live there. This leads to watery diarrhea, gas, and cramping.

Since one of the most common sugars in a baby's diet is lactose, a common strategy is to remove lactose in hope that it will slow down the diarrhea. Unlike standard infant formula, soy contains no lactose, making it a good temporary source of nutrition for babies with intestinal viral infections.

GOT GOAT'S MILK?

Does goat's milk have any role in the treatment of the fussy baby?
Although this may be Grandma's solution to colic, there are some good reasons why your infant shouldn't drink goat's milk. Used for many years as a cure-all for fussy babies, goat's milk was considered easier for babies to digest. Although it does form a softer curd in the stomach, it's not an appropriate source of nutrition for babies because of its unusual nutrient balance and high level of protein.

Specifically, goat's milk is deficient in vitamins B and C, folate, and iron. It contains levels of sodium, potassium, and protein that are too high for a baby's kidneys. Such concentrated levels of minerals can be life-threatening should a baby continue to drink it when sick or dehydrated. Despite its popularity with past generations, you shouldn't be using goat's milk or cow's milk with your baby under twelve months unless you happen to be a goat or a cow.

If goat's milk presents such a potential problem for babies, how come some people swear by it for allergy?

It may be that the babies that are being treated for "allergy" really have no problem with allergy. Again, allergy is often self-diagnosed and overdiagnosed, and is more often a problem of parental perception rather than a true immune problem. To the goat's credit, however, the softer curd formed by its milk may be enough to take the edge off of whatever nonallergic problem is making the babies fussy. So some babies may seem happier on goat's milk, but it's usually got nothing to do with allergy.

While it's true that most babies are able to drink goat's and cow's milk without showing any immediate problems, the risks of nutritional deficiencies, excessive protein load on the kidneys, and blood electrolyte imbalances make it a risky play. And just because a baby can drink something without becoming visibly ill doesn't mean it's an appropriate long-term source of nutrition.

My friend gave me a recipe for diluting goat's milk, which is supposed to make it safer for babies. Doesn't this take care of the concerns over excessive protein, salt, and so on?

The fact that some goat's milk advocates recommend dilution of goat's milk supports the belief that, in its raw form, it isn't appropriate for a baby's sensitive system. While dilution may make some of the concentrated minerals in goat's milk safer, it waters down certain nutrients, such as iron, vitamins A and C, and folate—nutrients that were deficient to begin with.

So to put the whole thing in a biblical context, "we're borrowing from Peter to pay Paul." We've brought the protein, sodium, and potassium levels down to an appropriate level for a baby but in turn have made it even less nutritious in terms of its vitamins. Sure, you can supplement with vitamins to make up what's been washed away, but it sure seems like a lot of work to make a baby tolerate something that nature didn't intend her to take. Stick with breast-feeding. If that doesn't work for you, use a nutritionally complete formula and save goat's and cow's milk for after twelve months.

WATCHING OUT FOR NUMBER TWO

How often does gas represent a formula problem?

If fixing gassy babies was as easy as making an extra trip to the grocery store, your pediatrician probably would have been out of business a long time ago. Gas is almost never a formula problem.

For those of us who think a lot about gas, we know that it comes from two sources: swallowed air and fermentation of sugars in the large intestine. Sugars present in the typical newborn diet are digested and absorbed in the small intestine, leaving very little available for fermentation and gas production by bacteria in the colon. Even if infant gas were a sugar absorption problem, it wouldn't correct itself with formula switching, since many of the formulas contain similar types of sugar. When gas disappears after a formula change, it's usually a coincidence or very wishful thinking.

Air swallowing, on the other hand, occurs very commonly in babies and typically is caused by excessive crying or difficulty feeding, perhaps due to the pain of reflux or an inappropriately sized nipple.

My three-month-old was recently begun on Nutramigen, a hypoallergenic formula, and his stools have become looser. Is this normal?

Yes. Casein hydrolysate formulas such as Nutramigen or Alimentum will cause a baby's stools to become slightly looser than those seen with standard infant formulas.

Does iron-supplemented infant formula cause constipation?

There is no evidence to support the widely held belief that iron-containing formulas lead to constipation in infants. Yes, the use of iron drops or pills leads to constipation in many people, but the amount of iron given in this way is many times higher than that found in formula.

The important thing to remember about infant formula is that the "added" iron simply provides what a baby needs for normal growth and really shouldn't be considered extra. In fact, formulas supplemented with iron should be considered regular, while nonsupplemented formulas should be regarded as low-iron preparations. If your baby doesn't get her iron through her formula, she'll have to get it some other way, which may be difficult, if not impossible, if solids haven't been started.

Iron is essential for the production of red blood cells, and a deficiency in iron is likely to lead to anemia by the age of six months. Several studies have suggested that iron deficiency during the first two years of life can lead to developmental delay. At particularly high risk are preemies, since the majority of a newborn's iron stores are established during the last trimester. For these reasons and more, low-iron infant formulas should have no place in infant nutrition.

What effect does soy formula have on a baby's bowel movement?

While you may look to soy formula as a fix for your baby's fussiness, you may wind up needing a fix for firm poop. Some parents have described mild constipation in babies on soy formula. If you find your baby straining more than normal and it's really critical that she feed with soy, you may try supplementing your baby with one to two teaspoons of dark corn syrup (found in your grocery store) mixed in three to four ounces of water twice a day.

Chapter 3

Breast-feeding

The jury is in. Breast-feeding is best for babies for so many reasons. And of all the decisions you'll make about feeding your baby, the decision to breast-feed may be the one that carries the longest consequences. I wrote in the introduction that there are very few things you can do to hurt your baby. While choosing not to breast-feed may not *hurt* your baby in the purest sense of the word, it's clear that it represents a compromise.

Unfortunately, breast-feeding failures are not always the fault of the mother or baby. Our healthcare system frequently fails the patients it's allegedly committed to serve, and it seems the deck is stacked against those mothers who choose to do what nature intended. Formal training in breast-feeding plays no part in many pediatric training programs, and where it exists it sits more as a token part of the training curriculum. The nutrition industry aggressively promotes the use of infant formulas among parents and pediatricians alike. Public breast-feeding is discouraged in subtle ways, and only recently have segments of corporate America begun to show signs of supporting breast-feeding employees.

Breast-feeding can be challenging and requires a firm commitment to see it through. While it shouldn't be seen as a personal failure, sometimes breast-feeding doesn't work. But more important, failing to breast-feed without good reason may represent a missed opportunity to provide your baby with the earliest advantage possible.

BREAST-FEEDING BASICS

Will my baby have to learn to breast-feed or will it be instinctive?

All healthy babies are born with an instinctive drive to suck, which is evident even minutes after they're born. You may notice that your baby "roots," or turns her head and opens her mouth when her lips are touched. This is a reflex that tells her to open wide for dinner. But while it may be instinctive for your baby, breast-feeding correctly requires a little support and coaching on your part. Look at yourself as someone who facilitates and monitors your baby's natural ability to feed.

Insist on the Breast

Nothing facilitates proper breast-feeding better than breast-feeding itself. Request that artificial nipples or pacifiers not be used. While you may be told that you "need your rest" and that an occasional bottle won't do any harm, this isn't necessarily the best advice. Few things promote a healthy start to breast-feeding than frequent exposure to the breast. The early experiences that a baby has help imprint in her mind what feeding is and should be.

Find a Quiet Place

When starting out, proper nursing requires a stress-free, quiet environment. The sights and sounds where you nurse will impact on your baby's ability to focus on feeding and your ability to relax and comfortably let-down. The proper environment sets the mood for the optimal feeding experience. While this may be difficult during your stay in the hospital, the staff are usually willing to provide quiet time with a sign on your door indicating that you're feeding.

Position Yourself and Your Baby

There are a number of ways to position yourself and your baby for breast-feeding, and you'll have to experiment to find what works for you. The most common nursing position is the cradle hold. This is what we typically envision when we think of the breast-fed baby. This involves "cradling" the child on your forearm with the head against your bent elbow and your hand supporting the bottom and thighs. This hold allows you to rotate your arm to position the baby properly facing your breast. When done correctly, the baby's whole body should be facing you and you should be chest to chest. A number of other nursing positions work well (in particular situations), depending upon your own needs and how your baby feeds. Be sure to speak with a lactation consultant to see what works best for you.

Establish a Proper Latch

While sucking may be instinctive, a proper latch (or attachment to the breast) requires your guidance. This is very important and is often the weakest link to successful feeding. An improper latch can lead to cracked, painful nipples, an unsatisfied baby, and poor feeding experience.

Once you're comfortable and you've positioned your baby in the vicinity of your breast, you're ready to help your baby latch on. While supporting your breast with your hand, stimulate her lower lip with your nipple in order to get her to open wide. This is often better done by trying to bring the baby to the nipple as opposed to pushing your nipple to the baby. Once your baby opens her mouth wide, take that opportunity to pull her toward you so that she grasps on to the entire nipple and then some. A correct latch should involve the entire nipple with an inch or so of surrounding areola and breast. Such a large area around the nipple is necessary because there are large ducts underneath the areola that store milk. These reservoirs are the source of milk when a baby sucks. When properly latched, a baby's jaws should be opened almost as wide as they can be, with the nose and chin touching the breast.

Be Patient

Understanding that breast-feeding requires patience and persistence at first is one of the key elements to helping your child learn to breast-feed properly. It may take four to six weeks before you and your baby are entirely comfortable with the process of breast-feeding. And just as babies need support and coaching, so do you. For those who have never breast-fed, ask to see a lactation consultant.

My baby is five days old and it seems that she wants to be on the breast every hour or two. Each feed is lingering into forty to forty-five minutes, and it seems like all I do is feed this child. Is this normal?

Frequent, protracted feeds are normal for breast-fed babies during the first couple of weeks of life. As frustrating as it may seem, frequent feeds ensure success through the stimulation of milk production and ultimately healthy weight gain. A newborn commonly spends up to forty-five minutes at a feed. Some of this time, of course, is spent sleeping, daydreaming, resting, and doing the things that newborns like to do. While it may seem like lollygagging, it's part of the adjustment to her outer world. Failing to allow infants to work through this period and adjust to the breast is one of the common roadblocks to breast-feeding.

Feeding patterns during this time period sometimes can be perceived as poor feeding or being "hungry all the time." No one wants his or her baby to be hungry, and consequently there's the temptation to top off with some formula. While this may seem like a good short-term solution to the situation, this in fact discourages your milk production and consequently undermines your ability to breast-feed appropriately over the long term. If you have questions about your particular situation that go beyond this, the best thing you can do is get the proper information from a lactation consultant.

Why the Breast Is Best

So you're not sure breast-feeding really makes a difference? Take a look at the facts:

BETTER NUTRITION AND DIGESTION

- Breast milk allows improved absorption or *bioavailability* of nutrients. Iron is nearly completely absorbed from breast milk; only about 10 percent of the iron in infant formula is absorbed.
- Breast milk naturally contains arachidonic and docosahexanoic acid, fatty acids suggested to improve visual and cognitive function in babies.
- Gastric emptying is faster in breast-fed infants. Factors naturally found in human milk stimulate motility and enhance maturity.

FEWER INFECTIONS

- Breast milk is a biologically active fluid containing immunoglobulins, lactoferrin, and lysozyme—all critical disease-fighting elements.
- Breast-fed babies are less likely to suffer from respiratory infections, ear infections, pneumonia, bronchiolitis, and bacterial meningitis.

FEWER DISEASES

- Breast-fed babies have a lower incidence of type-1 diabetes, Crohn's disease, celiac disease, lymphoma, and sudden infant death syndrome (SIDS).
- Babies at risk for asthma have been shown to have a reduced incidence and severity of lung symptoms later in life if breast-fed as infants.

IMPROVED INTELLIGENCE

- Long-term studies have shown small but measurable differences in intellectual performance in children breast-fed as infants.

BENEFITS FOR MOM

- Cost.
- Allows the uterus to contract back to its normal size after birth.
- Allows quicker return to your prepregnancy weight.
- Reduces the risk of ovarian cancer and, in premenopausal women, breast cancer.
- Delays the return of your menstrual period and may extend the time between pregnancies.

I'm small-chested and I'm concerned that I won't produce enough milk if I choose to breast-feed. Is this true?

It's rare that a woman motivated to breast-feed is unable to due to inadequately sized breasts. In fact, less than five percent of the population lacks the glandular tissue necessary for successful breast-feeding. You shouldn't make the decision to not breast-feed on this basis on your own. An exam by your physician or an experienced lactation consultant should help you determine whether this is an issue.

Signs that might indicate difficulty with adequate milk production include marked asymmetry of the breasts, limited changes in the breasts during pregnancy, and failure to see postpartum engorgement.

How will breast implants impact on my ability to breast-feed?

If you've had breast augmentation surgery, you're not alone. It's estimated that 1 to 2 million American women have breast implants. Unfortunately, the anticipated cosmetic benefits often outshadow the potential risks of future breast-feeding when the decision is made for surgery. Some surgeons often misrepresent, or even fail to mention, the potential impact of implants on breast-feeding. Fortunately, most women are able to breast-feed after implantation. When done properly, the surgery should involve no destruction of gland tissue, no interruption of milk ducts, and no interruption of innervation to the nipple—the most critical consequences of breast surgery.

It's important to consider the initial reasons for the augmentation—if a woman lacked functional breast tissue anyway, this alone may be a reason for breast-feeding difficulty and may be unrelated to the surgery itself. In a perfect world the adequacy of underlying breast tissue should be evaluated prior to surgery.

If you choose to breast-feed after having had breast implants, you probably should be monitored by an experienced lactation consultant. Engorgement can be a problem under these circumstances since the amount of free space available for the accumulation of milk is limited. This can lead to difficulty for the baby in expressing milk from the compressed ducts. Because of this, diaper counts, urine output, and weight should be followed closely. Frequent pumping is often recommended initially to minimize engorgement.

Do breast implants ever have to be removed? Despite the suggestion that silicone breast implants present a danger to those women who have opted for augmentation, they present no danger to breast-feeding infants. If you choose to breast-feed, it isn't necessary that they be removed and breast milk doesn't need to be monitored.

How will breast reduction surgery impact on my ability to breast-feed?

Unlike breast augmentation, breast reduction surgery tends to be more destructive since the replacement of the nipple, by definition, requires interruption of the ducts. It's very possible that if you've had breast reduction surgery you won't be able to breast-feed successfully. And even those women who are able to breast-feed are at a higher risk for impaired milk flow and subsequent infection. Be sure to discuss this with a lactation consultant before you make any decision regarding how you feed your child. Difficult feeding can occur for a number of reasons, including poor latch or awkward positioning, and in your case it may be unrelated to any prior surgery.

I have heard that breast milk is lower in iron than infant formula. Is this true?

While it's true that the level of iron in formula is much higher than that found in breast milk, it's important to understand what this really means. When we think about iron and babies, the most important thing to consider is not how much iron is in the baby's milk but rather how much is actually being absorbed. This is a concept that nutritional researchers refer to as *bioavailability*, and it's the true bottom line on nutrients and minerals. Under normal circumstances, the amount of iron absorbed from a variety of foods ranges from almost none to 20 percent; the rest is passed in our stool.

About 4 percent of the iron in fortified infant formula is absorbed compared to 50 percent of the iron in breast milk. This tenfold difference in absorption explains why formula manufacturers fortify their formulas to the extent that they do and illustrates that labels can be deceiving.

Is it true that breast-fed infants tend to be leaner than bottle-fed infants?

The big problem with studying the growth of breast-fed infants is the fact that so many breast-fed babies are supplemented with formula. This, of course, affects the outcome of any study since the babies aren't exclusively breast-fed and the degree of supplementation can vary tremendously. Keeping that in mind, studies have shown that the differences in growth between bottle-fed and breast-fed infants are minimal throughout the first three months of life but thereafter breast-fed infants tend to be leaner. In other words, they tend to weigh less for a given length when compared to bottle-fed infants. In the long run, there's no evidence that bottle-fed and breast-fed infants differ at all in their size.

I've heard that the growth of breast-fed babies needs to be followed on special growth curves. How do I know if my pediatrician is using them?

This really isn't accurate but deserves some explanation. In May of 2000 the U.S. Centers for Disease Control (CDC) released new pediatric growth charts for monitoring the growth of America's 82 million children. Unlike the previous charts available to physicians, which were essentially based on the growth patterns of formula-fed white kids, the new CDC charts reflect a more diverse population *including* breast-fed babies. These charts should be used by all physicians who see children.

Is it safe to breast-feed when I'm sick? How can I keep my baby from catching what I've got?

Breast-feeding mothers often worry about transmitting whatever they've got to their child. While it's good to make every effort possible to keep babies from getting sick, it's practically impossible to keep yourself clear of all illnesses—especially the common cold. Fortunately, Mom's cold or upper respiratory infection isn't a reason to avoid contact or stop breast-feeding. These illnesses aren't transmitted through breast milk. In fact, breast milk is naturally rich in immunoglobulins and infection-fighting cells that provide baby with the defense that her immune system can't yet provide. It's therefore critical that you *continue* to breast-feed when faced with an upper respiratory infection. Research shows that breast milk also may protect baby from otitis media (middle ear infection) and some gastrointestinal infections.

While you may not be able to safeguard baby entirely from catching your cold, common sense and good hygiene are probably the best defense. Remember that the most common viruses that cause colds are transmitted on the hands of infected people and the objects they've handled. Covering your mouth when you sneeze, strict hand washing, and limited exposure to sniffling strangers are probably the best measures against passing a bug on to your baby. Simply being close to baby, as in hugging or nursing, won't cause her to catch your cold. Don't wash or disinfect your breasts before nursing; the secretions and odor of the nipple are part of the sensation that babies like and associate with feeding.

How do I know if I'm producing enough milk for my baby?
The number of feeds and duration of feeding is a good indicator of how your baby is doing. Most breast-feeding infants early on will feed eight to twelve times in a twenty-four-hour period and spend thirty to forty-five minutes feeding. You should notice that your breasts are softer after a feed and that the baby seems satisfied.

Perhaps the best indicator that a baby is receiving sufficient breast milk is the presence of wet and dirty diapers. A breast-fed infant should produce eight or more wet diapers in a twenty-four-hour period and have at least one stool per day. Urination tells us that a breast-feeding baby's fluid intake is up to par and that her nutritional intake is most likely adequate. And no matter how much or how little any child takes, our goal is to make them grow. If they're growing, they're getting enough.

Is it possible for a mother to produce bad or inadequate breast milk?

For the mother of a baby having a hard time gaining weight, one of the first concerns is that her breast milk may not be good enough or rich enough. This is extremely rare. In fact, experts who deal with difficult breast-feeding cases consider this something so rare that it's worthy of report in the medical literature. Consequently, the analysis or testing of breast milk has no role in the practical management of breast-feeding.

Breast-feeding difficulties, especially those leading to growth problems, are most often the result of inadequate *volumes* of milk or poor *transfer* of that milk to the baby. This can occur due to any number of problems and requires the input of a good lactation consultant.

Why do breast-fed babies get jaundiced more easily?

Jaundice in breast-fed babies can occur early or late. *Early breast milk jaundice* occurs in the first few days after delivery and is usually a result of delayed maternal milk production. Limited fluid intake with diminished stimulation to stool frequently makes jaundice worse whether a child is bottle-fed or breast-fed. This is not a consequence of breast milk itself but rather the frequency or duration of feeding. Sometimes breast-fed children are supplemented with formula or water over the first day or two in order to maintain their hydration and in turn help improve their jaundice. As milk production improves so does their color.

Late breast milk jaundice usually peaks at one or two weeks of life. Unlike early breast milk jaundice, this unusual condition is believed to be the result of something inherent in the milk of some lactating women. A number of compounds have been identified in breast milk that may account for late breast milk jaundice, but none has been definitively linked as the true cause. Interestingly, among prior siblings of children with this condition, 70 percent also were jaundiced, suggesting that there is some genetic predisposition.

Does breast-feeding prevent obesity in children?

With all of the seemingly magical qualities of breast-feeding being discovered, it has been suggested that breast milk could serve as the cure for the latest obesity epidemic. And with nearly 6 million American children overweight, experts are looking earlier and earlier in life for a fix. Unfortunately, the studies looking at the role of breast-feeding in obesity are mixed. Some have demonstrated a protective effect while others have been inconclusive. This is a very difficult subject for clinical researchers to study since there are so many differences among breast-feeding mothers, such as their social backgrounds, length of breast-feeding, timing of solid introduction, and the use of supplemental formula. All of these variables are likely to influence a baby's ultimate body makeup and make scientific comparison and firm conclusions difficult if not impossible.

While the future may hold an answer to the breast-feeding–obesity question, an understanding of what's known may be the best defense against a tubby toddler. In children under the age of three, the greatest determinant of a baby's ultimate body type is that of her parents. Whether this represents genes or environment isn't entirely clear, but the message certainly could be construed that what goes for you also goes for your children. The environment and feeding attitudes you create for yourself may very well influence the adult your baby will one day become. With that it should be understood that breast-feeding represents the best option for facilitating an early start on a life of healthy eating whether it prevents obesity or not.

Is breast milk "brain food"?

If there is such a thing, breast milk appears to fit the bill. Numerous studies following a variety of neurodevelopmental outcomes have demonstrated small but statistically significant differences in breast-fed infants when compared with those fed formula. The most convincing and publicized study by Lucas in 1992 found a ten-point IQ advantage in a group of infants who had been followed from birth. While the evidence supporting improved intelligence is convincing, this is only one of a number of advantages conferred through breast-feeding.

I was recently found to be positive for the hepatitis C virus. Can I breast-feed?

Unfortunately, very little is known about the risk of hepatitis C virus transmission via breast milk. In fact, remarkably little is known about the transmission of hepatitis C from mother to baby in utero and at delivery. Despite the presence of hepatitis C genetic material in the breast milk of actively infected mothers, transmission to babies has never been proven. Most physicians are treating the hepatitis C breast-feeding issue on a case-by-case basis, and each mother has to determine what she's comfortable with. The Centers for Disease Control currently does not consider hepatitis C virus infection a contraindication to breast-feeding unless the mother has severe liver disease or coinfection with the HIV virus. The transmission of hepatitis C from mother to baby is a subject of active investigation, and new information is becoming available on a monthly basis.

Reasons Woman Shouldn't Breast-feed
Definite: HIV positive, active pulmonary tuberculosis, illegal drug use
Maybe: Hepatitis C positive

The other issue to consider here is whether you are considered to be actively infected with the hepatitis C virus. Just because you carry the antibody to the virus does not mean that your liver is necessarily infected or that you are contagious. The presence of the antibody suggests that your body has seen the virus at some time in the past. You may want to discuss this with your physician since further testing can be done to help sort this out.

If I pump and allow my baby to feed occasionally from a bottle, will she develop nipple confusion?

Everyone talks about nipple confusion when it comes to offering bottles to breast-fed babies. I'm not sure such a condition exists, since most babies aren't sophisticated enough to be confused about anything, and if they were going to be, it wouldn't be about how they want to eat. Most babies know what they want and when they want it when it comes to their milk. The difficulty a baby may experience in switching from breast to bottle has more to do with preference than any sort of confusion.

Should you choose to offer your child a bottle, any difficulties you have will be a result of (1) the personality characteristics of your baby, (2) the age at which you first introduce the bottle, and (3) the type of bottle system you choose to use.

With regard to personality, every baby is different, and their tolerance for change will vary dramatically. Some easygoing babies will have no problem taking breast milk directly from the source or through any type of bottle system. Other babies will be more discerning in their tastes and may insist on being fed exclusively from the breast. While the fickle baby may be trained, it's important to remember that how a baby prefers to feed has a lot to do with who she is.

The ability to feed from both the breast and bottle has a lot to do with the age at which a bottle is first introduced. Your best chances for ensuring that your baby will be able to feed both ways is to make sure that you don't offer the bottle too early or too late. Let your baby feed exclusively from the breast for the first three to four weeks to establish a clear feeling for the breast. At that point you can begin offering a bottle. One way to do this is to cut short your baby's feed by ten minutes or so and pass her on to her dad. The chances of feeding from an alternate source are always greater when the food is offered by someone who doesn't smell or feel like the baby's mom. Let her dad offer the bottle for the remaining time of the baby's feed.

Finally, the bottle system you choose may affect how well she can switch from breast to bottle. The way that milk is expressed from an artificial nipple is different from the way it's taken from the breast. Most artificial nipples require that suction be generated by the cheeks. This is very different from breast-feeding, where up-and-down movement of the jaw is the motion required for obtaining milk. Most babies learn to adapt, although some bottle systems such as the Avent® bottle system require the baby to use a jaw motion similar to that used on the breast. Unlike most systems, it requires that the infant take the entire nipple into the mouth much like breast-feeding. In most cases it isn't necessary to switch bottle systems, but it may make a difference with the discerning baby.

Do pacifiers have any impact on how babies breast-feed?

For the bottle-fed infant, the pacifier doesn't present too much of an issue, but it can be a problem for the breast-fed infant. Pacifiers, like bottles, can interfere with proper breast-feeding, and their use has been shown to be associated with early weaning. While you should be aware of the "risks" associated with pacifier use in your breast-fed infant, the ultimate decision is a personal one.

How early can I begin pumping my breasts?

Pumping your breasts can be useful for several different reasons. It allows you to prepare for feeding your baby in your absence and to remain comfortable at times when your production of milk isn't in sync with your baby's demand. Pumping also can serve a therapeutic role in the case of a breast infection or when one breast produces significantly more milk than the other.

There are no strict rules about when you can begin pumping your breasts. Some lactation consultants get concerned that women will overproduce milk if they pump, but that isn't necessarily true. It's very important that you remain comfortable, especially during the first few weeks after delivery.

Why do my breasts tingle sometimes when my baby cries?
This sensation represents let-down, or the release of milk, from the alveoli where milk is produced through the milk ducts and into the sinus areas where it can be expressed. While milk let-down typically is stimulated by suckling, certain visual or auditory stimuli can have the same effect. The hormone oxytocin, which is produced in the pituitary gland, is responsible for this reflex effect.

Why does my baby appear to prefer one breast to the other?
Breast-feeding mothers often report that their baby feeds very differently on each breast. In most cases this is nothing more than a curiosity but in others it creates a problem requiring the diagnostic skills of a lactation consultant.

Babies' physical problems related to pregnancy and delivery sometimes can make them prefer feeding on one side. Collarbone fractures from a difficult delivery or strained neck muscles due to positioning in the uterus can lead to pain in certain positions. Tongue-tied babies often are reported to have right- or left-handed preferences when it comes to feeding on the breast.

Differences in a mother's anatomy may be at the root of the problem. Women commonly will let-down milk differently in each breast due to natural anatomic differences in the breast ducts. Depending on the baby's feeding temperament, she may prefer a faster or slower flow of milk and select on that basis alone. Interestingly, some babies are mesmerized by the beating of their mother's heart and in turn favor the left breast.

Finally, a baby's preference may have nothing to do with her or her mother but rather the environment. If your nursery happens to have a fascinating visual attraction on one side and not the other, it could lead to a difference in how your baby feeds on that side. Young babies tend to do better when they have something to fix on. Once a child reaches a few months of age, however, these mesmerizing fixations will become a source of distraction and have the opposite effect.

Does a cesarian delivery have any impact on breast-feeding?

A cesarian delivery should have very little impact on your ability to breast-feed successfully. Most of the work to prepare your body for breast-feeding is done well before delivery. Studies have shown, however, that breast-feeding mothers who have undergone C-section are at higher risk for delayed milk production in the first few days after delivery. Whether this is due to the stress of surgery or physiologic differences in the type of delivery isn't clear. Depending on the events surrounding the delivery and the reason for C-section, early contact between baby and mother may not be possible. Such early bonding is felt to be a key factor in breast-feeding success. Irrespective of the way you deliver your baby, early input from an experienced lactation consultant should help to prevent problems before they develop.

Is it possible to breast-feed an adopted baby?

Yes, it is possible to breast-feed an adopted baby. This is referred to as *induced lactation*. Techniques for induced lactation may include stimulation of the breast and nipples for a few weeks prior to the anticipated adoption, very frequent feeding, use of a supplemental nursing system, and perhaps medications to help milk production. As one might imagine, bringing a mother who hasn't been pregnant to the point of completely nourishing her child is difficult and requires a great deal of work and commitment. It should be understood that, despite how hard you try, it may not be possible for you to nourish your child completely this way. Supplementation with formula or banked human milk is nearly always necessary at least for the first several weeks. This process obviously requires very close supervision by your pediatrician and an experienced lactation specialist to help maximize the chances of success and ensure the safety of your baby.

My daughter will be undergoing general anesthesia for a hernia repair. How many hours before the surgery will it be necessary that she not breast-feed?

While policies can vary from hospital to hospital, most require that breast-fed babies remain *NPO*, or nothing by mouth, for four to six hours before surgery. There is, however, literature to support that breast milk empties faster than formula from the stomach. Consequently some argue that children should be able to breast-feed up to three hours before surgery. Despite the evidence, most anesthesiologists prefer to err on the side of safety and require the traditional four- to six-hour waiting period.

I've just returned to work and if getting used to pumping around my workplace wasn't enough, I've been summoned for jury duty. Are breast-feeding mothers exempt?

Considering that exemptions exist for other less important activities, it seems that you should be. You'll only know, however, by inquiring with the court. A handful of states have enacted laws exempting breast-feeding mothers from jury commitment. Independent of legislation in this regard, many courts will make exemptions when your situation has been explained. Be sure to let them know about your baby's dependency on you as well as your degree of physical discomfort when unable to pump or feed.

Nursing on the Net

www.lalecheleague.org
Fantastic resource and a great place for information on breast-feeding. Up-to-date information on legislative activity in the different states.

www.breastfeeding.com
Comfortable layout and organization. Great cartoons and stories covering the lighter side of breast-feeding.

www.breastfeeding.org/law/maloney.html
A webpage including all the latest breast-feeding legislation maintained by Congresswoman Carolyn Maloney of New York.

While discreetly feeding my son in one of the common areas of the mall recently, I was approached by one of the nearby shop owners and told that breast-feeding wasn't allowed. Is this right?

This is wrong. Women have the right to breast-feed in public in the same way that they can bottle-feed. While some states have enacted legislation regarding public breast-feeding, this serves not to legalize it but rather to emphasize a woman's right to feed where and when necessary for her baby. Despite how angry you may be about the welcome you receive as a breast-feeding mother, remember that defiance isn't the way to change attitudes about breast-feeding.

Keep in mind that breast-feeding and other activities that are also our right may not be appropriate in all settings. As natural as breast-feeding may be, not everyone may be interested in sharing the nurturing relationship you have with your baby. Be respectful of those around you, and people will usually reciprocate. For more information on your rights as a breast-feeding mom and new legislation in your state, check out *www.lalecheleague.org*

EATING AND SLEEPING

My baby often falls asleep after feeding from one breast, leaving my other breast painfully engorged. What should I do?
The problem of the sleepy baby is common and is usually the result of individual sleeping patterns, overstimulation, swaddling, and caretaking routines. Early on in a baby's life, the effects of epidural medication need to be considered, but we'll assume that's not the issue in this case. While the engorged breast may seem (and feel!) like the most pressing issue, the biggest concern here is whether the baby is getting enough milk. You should assess this with diaper counts. Assuming that you're comfortable with the baby's intake and hydration, you can then consider the details of stimulating the somnolent baby for better feeding. Try the following changes:

- *Avoid keeping the baby too wrapped up.* Cozy, swaddled babies are more inclined to snooze than look for food. Keep your baby loosely wrapped during feeding and allow some contact with your skin. Try putting your baby down unwrapped for a couple of minutes before completing the feed on the first breast. Perhaps change her diaper and let her rouse a bit. This may help stimulate her to finish her feeding.

- *Feed the baby before she becomes too hungry.* Exhausted babies like to sleep when they find someplace warm to settle. Try to intercept and feed when cues such as rooting and hand sucking indicate hunger.
- *Keep your baby awake with a steady flow of milk.* Once your baby slows down or shows signs of dropping off, the stimulation offered through gentle hand expression may stimulate her to keep going. You can also achieve this by offering a little milk through a dropper or via a supplemental nursing system.
- *Burp in the sitting position.* When you put your baby over your shoulder, she's apt to want to cuddle and drift off to sleep.

If you're still painfully engorged, pump or hand express only a few minutes for comfort and store the milk for later use. Start your baby on this fuller breast at the next feed and alternate if necessary.

This is, interestingly, one of the rare circumstances in pediatrics where a parent will complain about their baby sleeping.

Is it reasonable to try to get my baby on a regular three-hour schedule? I've heard that it's good to try to start this early.
Scheduling your baby for feeds shouldn't be a priority. If it happens, great. But don't expect much before the first three to four weeks. During this time it's very important that a

---

Fact or Fiction: Nursing Your Baby to Sleep Will Make Her Dependent on Nursing for Sleep

Fiction. Considering that babies spend the majority of their day either sleeping or eating, it stands to reason that your baby may very well fall asleep after a feed. This is entirely normal. Furthermore, many very normal, well-adjusted babies feed shortly before going down for the evening. The suggestion that your child will become dependent on certain comfort measures for sleep is false.

Fact or Fiction: Babies Are Incapable of Regulating Their Own Hunger Patterns and Need Parents to Do It for Them

Fiction. Babies do not need to have their hunger patterns regulated. In fact, babies do a very good job of listening to their bodies and asking for what they want when they need it. What parents often don't understand is that a baby's drive to eat isn't based on the social cues, pressures, and emotional factors that dictate an adult feeding schedule. The false notion that we can manipulate or control a baby's appetite and metabolism is based on our desire to make a newborn fit *our* schedule and needs. A baby's feeding pattern should be based on her natural needs rather than what's most convenient for other members of the household.

---

baby learn to nurse on demand both to provide the necessary nutrition and hydration as well as to stimulate your production of milk. There may be some points in the day when she will want to feed every hour. This is normal and should be encouraged since this is likely her active time. (You may notice that her active times may correspond with her periods of activity when she was in utero.)

After the first few weeks you may find you and your baby falling into some regular schedule, which should be a natural process rather than one that's planned. During this time the give-and-take reciprocity of breast-feeding is unfortunately weighted in favor of your baby. What's convenient for her will likely not be convenient for you or your schedule. Don't be discouraged. That will change. You'll find that your baby's schedule and demands ultimately will be predictable enough for your PalmPilot.

My daughter is eight months old and still doesn't sleep through the night. She's advancing well on solids and has always breast-fed exclusively. Is it possible that she isn't getting enough and would benefit from formula supplementation?

By eight months old your child should be able to sleep through the night without a problem. And despite the fact that she'll take the breast at that hour doesn't necessarily mean that she's hungry. This more likely represents a learned behavior based on eight months of experience. Children at this age often awaken on their own to find themselves alone and frightened, and they'll always welcome company.

As hard as it may seem, you'd be best off to try to extinguish this pattern earlier rather than later. The best approach may be to terminate nighttime visits cold turkey. If you must offer some consolation during the transition, send your partner so that a midnight feed won't be expected. Make the visit short and sweet with as little close interaction as possible. These visits should become shorter and shorter as you let her work it out on her own. Ultimately the goal should be for you, and your baby, to sleep peacefully through the night in your respective beds.

My three-month-old is beginning to sleep through the night and my breasts become uncomfortably engorged toward early morning. Is there anything I can do for this?

Unfortunately, there's no magic solution, and all of your options involve getting out of bed. You can either pump or wake your baby up to feed. Most mothers would prefer to let sleeping babies lie and choose to pump. You may be able to get through the night by pumping immediately before going to bed. Keep in mind that while having a baby sleep through the night is a frequently sought-after goal by many mothers, long periods of time without feeding has been associated with the early return of menses in the breast-feeding mother.

Fact or Fiction: Cabbage Leaves Help to Relieve Engorged Breasts

Probably fact (depending on how engorged you are). This frequently recommended home-brew therapy, which involves the placement of leaves directly on the breast, has been reported to relieve the pain of breast engorgement commonly experienced during the first week after delivery. While it's unknown why this effect occurs, many respected lactation specialists swear by its effectiveness. Unfortunately, cabbage leaf research isn't considered a priority. What few clinical studies have been done have been inconclusive.

Does this mean you shouldn't give it a try? Absolutely not. Try rolling out cabbage leaves to make them pliable and place them between you and a bra large enough to fit a small salad. Keep them there until they wilt. If you don't get any relief from your engorgement within two days, see your doctor.

Fact or Fiction: Lactation Consultants Are Heavily Biased in Favor of Attachment Parenting Theories and Are Thus Against Any Type of Routine Feeding

Fiction and fact. While not all lactation consultants can be labeled as attachment parenting advocates, all responsible lactation consultants should be against structured, routine feeding early on. In fact, any lactation consultant or physician who advocates early structured feedings for the breast-fed baby should be considered suspect. The metabolic needs of infants normally change from time to time, making nutritional demand variable. More simply put, babies go through growth spurts and other changes that make schedules impractical for their nutritional needs.

Breast-feeding mothers normally are spared their periods until weaning due to the effect of hormones involved in lactation. Most nonnursing mothers, in contrast, are menstruating by the third month postpartum.

If you prefer not to pump, remember that breast-feeding is a two-way street traveled by both mother and baby—asking your child to help keep you comfortable isn't unreasonable, even at 3 A.M.

EATING FOR TWO

How safe are alcohol and caffeine for breast-feeding mothers?
After nine months of disciplined abstinence, you may be ready for that first cool glass of Chablis. And so long as you're aware of when enough's enough, the occasional use of alcohol shouldn't present a problem for you or your baby. While studies done in a clinic setting have shown slightly decreased volumes of feeding in babies shortly after maternal alcohol exposure, the sedating effect may be helpful in some mothers. Despite how relaxing it may be, mothers should avoid breast-feeding for two hours after drinking. This should ensure that your baby's level of alcohol exposure is minimized. Peak alcohol levels are noted in milk about thirty to sixty minutes after consumption by itself. When taken with food it's a little longer.

Fact or Fiction: Drinking Beer Will Enhance Milk Production

This is unclear. Modern folklore tells us that moderate consumption of beer by lactating women may be beneficial for breast-feeding success. It is clear that there is a component of beer that can stimulate prolactin secretion and enhance milk production. It appears that this component is not alcohol but rather a sugarlike substance from barley. Consequently, the effect of beer on prolactin production is also seen with nonalcoholic beer. Unfortunately, no well-designed clinical studies have been done to study the effects of beer on milk production.

While it's possible that the sedating effect of alcohol (independent of the barley effect) may be beneficial to the breast-feeding mother, it isn't recommended during breast-feeding. An occasional beer is fine, but don't count on it for breast-feeding success.

What about discarding milk that you've expressed after a drink or two? Don't waste your time. There's no sense in pumping and discarding milk after drinking since milk levels match blood levels. In other words, alcohol isn't stored in milk. When the blood level goes down, so does the level in milk.

Concerning caffeine, the same commonsense, everything in moderation approach will most likely serve you best. Unlike alcohol, very little caffeine is passed into a mother's milk. However, the caffeine that does make it through to the milk can accumulate over the short term in a baby's body and have similar stimulating effects.

I've heard that my avoiding dairy products while breast-feeding will keep my baby from becoming fussy and irritable. Is this true?

The recommendation that dairy products be withheld for the colicky baby is a long-standing practice. Unfortunately, what's commonly practiced and what's been proven are often very different. There is no evidence that restricting a mother from cow's milk protein has any impact on a baby's behavior. We know that proteins in a mother's diet are often expressed in her milk and up to 5 percent of newborns have some degree of milk protein hypersensitivity. So it stands to reason that some percentage of colicky breast-fed babies would respond to this.

Whether there are studies to back it up or not, what you choose to believe is probably more important than what's been proven. Many women swear by this practice, and probably just as many pediatricians promote it. And like so many other methods in medicine, if it fits the can't-hurt, might-help category, it's worth a try. If you choose to forgo dairy products and notice a positive change, you may consider a challenge with the reintroduction of dairy products in four to eight weeks. This will either confirm your suspicion or prove that dairy has got nothing to do with your baby's behavior and free you to eat as you wish.

If you choose a dairy-free diet and it seems to do the trick, be sure to talk to your physician about the possible need for a calcium supplement. It's possible that the calcium in your bones could be sacrificed to provide adequate calcium in your baby's milk.

Can breast-fed babies be allergic to mother's milk?

I never like to tell mothers that their baby is allergic to their milk. More tactfully put, a baby may be allergic to proteins in the mother's diet expressed in her milk. Almost universally, allergic symptoms disappear when the common offending antigens are removed from the diet.

One of the most common signs of allergy in the breast-fed infant is the presence of blood and mucus in the stool. This allergic colitis is the result of contact between foreign protein (most often cow's milk protein) with the lining of

---

Fact or Fiction: The Foods You Eat While Breast-feeding Could Set Your Child Up for Later Food Allergies

For families at high risk for allergy and eczema, this is true. Studies have shown that mothers who excluded highly allergenic foods from their diets while breast-feeding had children with significantly less eczema and food allergy when compared with children of mothers with unrestricted diets. These differences, however, have not been found to extend beyond toddlerhood. So for the vast majority of the population, an unrestricted diet while breast-feeding shouldn't raise concerns unless you come from a high-risk family. And even then the long-term impact appears to be minimal.

the intestine. It is a temporary condition of infancy with most babies showing no difficulty after six or eight months of age. Wheezing, hives, congestion, and vomiting represent a less frequently seen type of reaction that often requires closer monitoring and longer restriction from the offending protein.

My four-week-old recently developed painful bowel movements with blood and mucus. I've been told by his pediatrician that this represents a milk protein allergy and to restrict my intake of foods with milk protein. How restrictive do I need to be?

Mothers are always looking for specifics when it comes to milk protein restrictions for their allergic babies. And as if you haven't made enough compromises in your own diet, the idea of limiting dairy products can be challenging in a number of ways. Unfortunately, casein and whey, the culprits responsible for milk protein colitis in babies, are found in a variety of foods. Some of those foods, such as milk and butter, are obvious, while things like chocolate and caramel coloring may come as a surprise.

To complicate matters, every child has a different degree of sensitivity, and a complete restriction may not be necessary in your case. You may start with restriction of the major sources of milk protein and see how your baby improves

---

Milk Protein Sources

COMMON SOURCES

butter	cottage cheese	half-and-half
casein and whey	curd	hydrolysates (milk, casein, whey)
artificial butter flavor	custard	nougat
caseinates	pudding	sour cream
cheese	ghee (clarified butter)	yogurt

LESS OBVIOUS MILK PROTEIN SOURCES

margarine	chocolate	nondairy creamer (check for casein)
deli meats	high protein flour	brown sugar flavoring

SOURCE: ADAPTED FROM K. HENDRICKS, C. DUGGAN, AND W. A. WALKER, *THE MANUAL OF PEDIATRIC NUTRITION*, 3RD ED. (LONDON: B. C. DECKER, 2000).

over one to two weeks. Remember that it takes a few days to clear your breast milk from offending proteins and a couple of weeks to heal the colon. If there is still occasional blood or mucus, you may look at your diet for some of the less common sources. Talk to your doctor to see how strict you need to be.

Can spicy food in my diet make my breast milk spicy?

Yes, the food you eat can change the flavor of your breast milk. It takes approximately four to six hours from the time you eat a food for its flavor to appear in your milk. The fact that babies can experience so many different taste sensations before ever making it to the table is one of the things that make breast-feeding so special. In fact, there's some evidence to suggest that the early exposure enjoyed by breast-fed babies leads to broader taste preferences as toddlers.

Do breast-fed babies need extra vitamins?

Generally speaking, healthy, full-term, breast-fed infants rarely need any sort of vitamin supplementation. However, breast milk does contain very little active vitamin D. Because of this, babies with dark skin who receive very little exposure to the sun are recommended to take a supplement. Sun exposure, on the order of a few minutes a day, is critical in converting the dietary form of vitamin D to the active form used by the body.

Iron tends to be a nutritional sore spot among breast-fed infants. While the demands for iron after six months often exceed what breast milk has to offer, most infants compensate with their intake of cereal and other iron-containing foods. Certainly the breast-fed child who hasn't advanced onto solids by this age should be considered for an iron supplement.

Independent of a baby's source of nutrition, fluoride supplementation should be considered after the age of six months depending on the content in your local water supply. Breast milk does contain small amounts of fluoride that tend to reflect that level. So even if your baby doesn't consume your tap water directly, the exposure through your breast milk may be enough to warrant withholding supplementation. Excessive fluoride exposure in children can lead to a condition called fluorosis, which is characterized by a mottled discoloration of the tooth enamel.

Does my breast-fed baby need fluoride supplementation if I'm drinking tap water that contains fluoride?

While fluoride was once pushed without thought, we're now aware of the risks associated with extra intake. Fluoride is expressed in breast milk in small amounts, and its levels reflect your intake. Given its unpredictable levels in breast milk, don't rely on what you drink to provide him with what he needs. If your child is over six months old and you are breast-feeding exclusively, he should be receiving a fluoride supplement. If you drink a significant amount of water, bottled or nonfluoridated water is recommended in order to minimize the risk of excessive fluoride exposure in your baby.

How long can breast milk be frozen?

Expressed breast milk should be frozen within forty-eight hours of expression and may be safely stored in the freezer section of a refrigerator freezer for three to four months and in a deep freezer (0 degrees F) for several months. When defrosting, thaw rapidly in warm water. *Never* use a microwave, since this may break down certain nutrients. Once milk is thawed, it should be used within twenty-four hours and should never be refrozen.

I'm currently on antibiotics for a sinus infection. Is it OK to breast-feed?

You need to depend on your physician to determine what's safe for you and your baby given your particular infection. Given the vast number of antibiotics available on the market and the small number of infections that respond to one drug only, it's unusual that breast-feeding needs to be discontinued on the basis of an antibiotic choice. When this situation does come up, however, breast-feeding often can be withheld temporarily during the time of treatment. If you're uncertain about the safety of a medication you've been prescribed, a good lactation consultant should be able to offer the reassurance you need or intercept when a medication may have been improperly dispensed.

Some Common Antibiotics

Sulfa: Sulfa drugs shouldn't be used during the first month of life because they interfere with the binding of bilirubin to proteins in the blood. This can result in the worsening of a baby's jaundice. Exposure of a baby to any sulfa medication can result in a sensitization reaction if there's a strong family history of sulfa allergy.

Erythromycin: Erythromycin drugs tend to be OK although they can interfere with the metabolism of other medications, especially seizure and heart medications. Erythromycin may be contraindicated if either you or your baby are taking other medications like these.

Cephalosporins: Most cephalosporin medications (often contain "ceph" in their names) are considered safe during breast-feeding, although they are commonly reported to cause diarrhea.

Flagyl: Flagyl (metronidazole) is an antibiotic commonly used for vaginal and gastrointestinal infections. Its levels in breast milk approach that found in the mother's blood, making it a contraindicated medication for breast-feeding mothers. Unfortunately, some of the infections treated with Flagyl respond to no other medication, making it a necessity in some cases. In some infections it is effective as a single, large dose, which requires that a baby be withheld from the breast (with milk expressed and discarded) for only a day or so. Ask your physician about this in the event that you need Flagyl.

When using antibiotics as a breast-feeding mother, you need to be concerned about the risk of thrush, a word commonly used to describe the oral yeast infection found in babies. It appears as a cheesy white deposit on the lining of a child's cheek and tongue, and it can lead to irritability and poor feeding. Once infected, a mother's nipples can become colonized, leading to reinfection or chronic seeding of a baby's mouth after treatment. In the event of recurrent oral thrush, or sometimes after a single episode, often the mother is treated with antifungal medications by mouth and with medication applied to the breast and nipple.

Is dieting prohibited while breast-feeding?
While working to reestablish your prepregnancy figure may be a priority, remember that you're eating for two and any shortcomings in your nutrition are likely to affect either you or your baby. Also keep in mind that breast-feeding will naturally keep you lean—you should expect to drop about one to two pounds a month for the first few months. With that said, dieting should not be a consideration while breast-feeding. Put the health of you and your baby first, let nature do its thing, and wait until weaning before considering diets.

How safe is a vegetarian diet for breast-feeding mothers?
A nursing infant isn't getting all the nutrients he needs through the breast if his mother is not well nourished. What a baby receives is often a reflection of what Mom eats (or doesn't eat). If you eat dairy products and eggs, you shouldn't have a problem. Calcium and vitamin D supplements are usually recommended for nursing vegan mothers to reduce a baby's risk of developing rickets as well as to maintain your own nutrient stores. Exclusively breast-fed infants of strict vegetarian mothers also can be at risk of vitamin B12 deficiency. If you follow a strict vegetarian diet, it's wise to take a multivitamin supplement. If you're opposed to taking vitamin supplements, you can get adequate amounts of B12 through fortified soy milk or cereal products, sufficient vitamin D through normal sunlight exposure, and proper calcium by eating lots of leafy green vegetables, such as broccoli and kale, and nuts, such as almonds and hazelnuts. Tofu and blackstrap molasses are excellent sources of calcium as well.

If you're a strict vegetarian who isn't breast-feeding or if you anticipate weaning in the near future, you can give baby a soy-based infant formula, which provides a sound nutritional alternative to breast milk and standard formula and contains no animal products. Do not substitute homemade mixtures or soy milk for commercial infant formula or breast milk.

I have heard that pesticides from the fruits and vegetables I eat can make their way into my breast milk. Is this true and do I need to have my milk tested?

Exposure to environmental pollutants is inevitable considering that we as humans tend to feed from the top of the food chain. Toxins present in the environment tend to concentrate the farther up the food chain you go, and most toxins tend to concentrate in fat. And considering the high concentration of fat in breast milk, it isn't hard to see how pollutants can concentrate there.

Despite the fact that chemical residue is known to be found in human milk, it is rarely ever a reason to rule out breast-feeding. The potential benefits of breast-feeding far outweigh any effect from environmental contaminants, and problems have been reported only in cases where there's been significant toxic exposure by the mother.

Considering that there are no accepted standards for breast milk testing and little is known about what is considered safe, screening should be restricted to a research setting.

If I'm breast-feeding, can I eat honey?

Yes. While honey should not be given to babies under a year due to the potential risk for neonatal botulism, typically adults are unaffected. Botulinum toxin is not passed through the breast milk.

How safe are cold and allergy medications during breast-feeding?

Given the popularity of over-the-counter cold preparations for stuffy noses, this is a very common question. The situation with cold medications tends to be less of a problem since their use is usually short term and often not a necessity. Allergy medications, on the other hand, present an issue year-round for many women.

Most allergy medications fit into a category of medications called antihistamines. Histamine is the chemical released by cells in the body that react to environmental allergens. By suppressing the effects of histamine, allergic symptoms can typically be controlled. The allergy control achieved with this class of medicine comes with a cost, however, since many antihistamines have the potential to make you drowsy.

And what few people realize is that while antihistamines can cause drowsiness in adults, babies can become jittery and tremulous with significantly altered sleep patterns. A mother who's expecting a groggy baby often overlooks these symptoms. And the effect of antihistamines isn't limited to the baby. Antihistamine medications tend to dry out mucous membranes and sometimes can slow a mother's milk production. This effect tends to vary from mother to mother and shouldn't be a reason for avoiding their use unless production becomes a problem.

In general, any antihistamine used should be taken immediately *after* a breast feed in order to minimize the levels of the medication in the milk. This strategy is more difficult with the newer-generation, long-acting antihistamines that are taken only once or twice a day. These medications tend to maintain a higher continuous level in the mother's bloodstream. There's very little information on antihistamine concentrations in breast milk, and antihistamines should be used with caution.

Concerning cold preparations, combination over-the-counter products should be avoided if at all possible since these products can contain alcohol, aspirin, or any number of other additives that may not be optimal for baby. Considering that the effects of most cold medicines is, at best, marginal, it may be best to avoid these altogether. If you must, pseudoephedrine is considered safe for breast-feeding by the American Academy of Pediatrics. Acetaminophen and ibuprofen are compatible with breast-feeding and may be all you'll need.

WATCHING OUT FOR NUMBER TWO

What's the normal number of dirty diapers for a breast-fed infant?
Dr. Marianne Neifert (Dr. Mom) tells her patients that after four days, a baby should be having four stools per day for at least four weeks. Dr. Mom's "rule of fours" has plenty of exceptions but still touches nicely on the bowel pattern of the breast-fed baby.

The first few days of life a normal breast-fed infant may have fewer than four stools per day—this is a function of how much milk a mother is producing. A baby's meconium (the thick black material passed after birth) should be gone within forty-eight hours after birth, and your colostrum will act as a natural laxative to help this along. Once into the routine of feeding, the first month of life is marked by at least four to six yellow, seedy stools per day. Beyond a month or two it isn't uncommon for breast-fed infants to stool only once daily or every other day. This probably has to do with the maturity of intestinal squeezing patterns and changes in the bacteria of the colon.

My four-day-old passes one stool a day that's very black and tarry like the day she was born. Is this normal?
No. Your baby's meconium (the tarry black stuff passed after birth) should be gone by about forty-eight hours of life. We'll allow transitional stools on days two to three but certainly by day 4 she should be well on her way to the seedy mustardy yellow stool of the healthy breast-fed infant. The concern here is that your baby isn't receiving enough milk. Have her weighed and evaluated immediately by your physician.

Is it normal for my baby to have a dirty diaper every time he feeds?

**Fact or Fiction: Breast-fed Infants Use
More Diapers than Bottle-fed Infants**

While diaper usage shouldn't influence how you feed your baby, breast-fed infants do in fact have more bowel movements. This difference is more pronounced earlier in life. By four months most infants, regardless of how they're fed, pass an average of two stools per day. Why the breast-fed infant produces stools more frequently than nonbreast-fed infants isn't exactly known. This difference is perhaps due to alterations in colonic bacteria as well as factors in human milk that help promote intestinal squeezing.

Yes, this is entirely normal, and it's referred to as the *gastrocolic reflex*. When the stomach is distended, the colon is stimulated to squeeze, thereby producing a poop. It is most pronounced during the first couple of months of life and diminishes with time.

I've heard that breast-fed infants never get constipated. Is this true?

Never say never. While breast milk may be the perfect food, breast-fed infants are prone to neurological and anatomical abnormalities just like formula-fed babies. Remember that when we're discussing constipation, we're talking about difficulty in being able to pass a stool, not necessarily the frequency of the bowel movement. Breast-fed infants beyond the first couple of months of age can go a few days between movements and not have any problem. Any recurring screaming, grunting, or pulling up of the legs without the production of a stool should be evaluated by your physician.

WEANERS

How long do I need to breast-feed in order to give my baby the advantage of breast milk?

At the risk of sounding evasive, as long as possible. The many advantages provided by breast milk represent a continuum depending on how long it's available to a child—the longer a child is breast-fed, the greater the likelihood that she'll benefit from all of its wonderful attributes. With respect to brain development, for example, research has suggested that the greater the total volume of milk taken by a baby (i.e., the longer a child is breast-fed), the higher the scores of neurodevelopmental outcome. The infection-fighting properties of human milk are dependent on the presence of the mother's valuable immunoglobulins at the time an infection tries to take hold. So the ability to fight off the more common intestinal infections faced during the first year or two of life is really a function of whether the child is breast-fed at the time of exposure. The longer you breast-feed, the better off your baby is likely to be.

My child is six months old and I'm interested in weaning him to formula. My girlfriends have all breast-fed their babies well beyond nine months and they make me feel so guilty. Am I really doing something wrong?

Great job for making it to six months! You've done better than the majority of American women who start breast-feeding. You've also given your child a great start, and the advantages that you've conferred through six months of breast-feeding will, it is hoped, follow her for a long time.

While social support networks are a key element to breast-feeding success, there can be conflict when your opinion about length of feeding or weaning differs with that of your friends or support network. In fact, the competition among some mothers would almost seem to qualify breast-feeding as a contact sport. While it's good to have role models, the decision of when and how to wean should be a closely held decision between you and your baby and it should never involve guilt. The issues facing you at home and in the workplace may be very different from those of your friends, and you've got to make the decision that's right for you. Don't let the concept of superior motherhood affect either the feeding relationship with your child or the relationship with your friends. And remember, friends don't force friends to breast-feed.

I'll be returning to work in a few weeks and I've heard that I should probably just pump and feed my baby from a bottle so she doesn't get used to me and my breast. Is this valid?

The urgency of a baby to adopt bottle-feeding is an invalid myth commonly promoted among daycare centers. While it may be easier for them to have a well-trained bottle-fed student in their class, this may not be what's best for your child. Going back to work and the fear of potentially alienating your child shouldn't prevent you from initiating breast-feeding. And going back to work doesn't mean that you can't have the close emotional bond that both you and your baby derive from feeding at the breast.

Keep in mind that if you choose to feed your child breast milk exclusively by bottle from the start, you're unlikely to be able to feed her from the breast over the long term. The type of nipple an infant prefers, be it artificial or natural, is determined in the first several weeks of life. And a child who is fed primarily from the breast has an easier time transitioning to an occasional bottle than the exclusively bottle-fed infant has going back to the breast. It's just the way babies are.

My baby is six weeks old and won't take milk from a bottle. I'll be returning to work in a few weeks and I need to make this transition. Any advice?

This is an anxiety-provoking scenario for a lot of mothers who are forced to balance work and breast-feeding. But don't despair; this is usually a temporary problem and one that requires nothing more than a little adjusting on your baby's part. Consider the following tips to help with the transition:

- *Let someone else feed the baby at first.* Your odor, sound, and touch will make the baby's preference for the real thing all that more powerful. Try to recruit someone else to introduce the bottle. Be sure to encourage him or her to cuddle, make eye contact, and talk to the baby in a way you normally would while feeding. Once a stable pattern of feeding from the bottle has been established, you'll be able to bottle-feed on your own.

- *Use expressed milk in the bottle.* If you intend to wean to infant formula, be sure to use your own milk at first so as not to make the transition too extreme. Once the bottle has been accepted, a different milk may be tried.
- *Feed in a different position.* Sometimes a different perspective will facilitate a different type of feeding.
- *Feed while walking around.* As with so many other problems in young babies, the rhythmic motion of walking or rocking sometimes will distract the baby from the issue at hand.
- *Try different nipples at different temperatures.* Sometimes a baby's reluctance has to do with the quality and texture of the nipple you've provided. If your baby has to work too hard to feed, or if the nipple provides much more than what she's used to, it could lead to a difficult transition. Sometimes the sensation of a different nipple temperature, such as one that's been in the refrigerator, will make a difference.

Is there a special formula that should be used when weaning a baby from the breast?

If you wean your baby from the breast before the end of the first year, she'll need to be provided with an infant formula. Despite rumors and old wives' tales about what's best for the weaning baby, the type of formula makes no difference to the otherwise healthy infant.

My son has mild reflux, and it seems as if it became worse when I weaned to formula. Is this possible?

Yes, this is entirely possible. Babies with reflux frequently will take a couple of steps backward when they wean from the breast. This is due to the fact that breast milk empties more efficiently from the stomach than manufactured formulas. Delayed emptying of the stomach is one of the handful of problems that lead babies to have reflux to begin with, and the effects of breast milk are often what helps them keep

it all together. Increased spitting on formula is by no means
a given, and it probably shouldn't factor into your weaning
decision *unless* your child happens to have moderate to severe reflux. In most circumstances, however, any increase in
the spits will represent more of an inconvenience to you
than a threat to your child.

What is a nursing strike?

A nursing strike is the baby's sudden refusal to nurse. While
temporary, a nursing strike can occur anytime and is sometimes the result of maternal factors such as the onset of
menses, changes in soap or perfume, or dietary changes.
While many mothers take a strike personally, it may be the
result of infant health factors, such as teething, ear infection,
or thrush. Before taking the matter to heart, take your baby
to the doctor to have these issues checked out.

Otherwise consider increasing the amount of personal attention you give to your baby while feeding. Feed in a quiet
place and offer more cuddling and stroking. Consider offering the breast while walking around. Once latched, sit down
in a new area with new visual cues. Sometimes sharing a
bath will offer the baby a chance to latch. Typically, striking
babies will begin to nurse when it's their choice. Until then,
don't be afraid to pump in the face of painful engorgement
and don't interpret a nursing strike as an effort to "self-wean."

My son has been breast-feeding exclusively for seven months. We have tried to begin weaning to a bottle but he's not interested. What can we do?

Some breast-feeding advocates would say that this indicates
he's a genius. While that may be the case, there's unfortunately very little you can do. If a baby hasn't fed from a bottle by this age, he's unlikely to pick it up. Your best bet may
be to try to transition to a tippy cup. You may notice that at
this age babies observe what you do with a cup. In fact, they
may want to model what you do and even drink from the
same cup you're using. If you're fortunate enough to have a
child as adventurous as this, simply offering breast milk in a

---

Fact or Fiction: The Appearance of Teeth Means It's Time to Wean

For those unfamiliar with breast-feeding, it would seem that teeth represent a painful red flag to wean, but for the baby with good technique, nothing could be further from the truth. A proper latch involves a wide-open mouth and a proper suck should involve nothing resembling a bite. While breast-feeding moms will report an occasional nip while initiating a latch or coming off the breast, this shouldn't influence your decision to wean.

---

tippy cup at the next feed may be all it takes. If he refuses, you may need to (1) give in and decide that the two of you aren't quite ready for this step, (2) offer milk from a regular cup in the hope that the novelty will allow him to transition to a tippy cup, or (3) let him cry it out during one feed a day in the hope that he'll give in and take it.

I have been breast-feeding my daughter for nearly two and a half years. Any tips on weaning her?

Weaning is hard on everyone involved, and there's no one approach that's going to make it easier. With that, you should approach weaning your daughter just as you would a baby at any age. Gradually drop off feeds on a weekly basis, saving perhaps her nighttime and morning feeds for last. Consider letting Dad take over bedtime to ease the temptation to feed. If the morning feed seems to be the holdout, be sure to have breakfast made so solid food and nutritious snacks are available as a diversion. Sometimes the key to weaning at this age is more attention and T.L.C. to make up for the perceived loss on your and your daughter's part.

To make things easier for everyone at this point, you might also want to consider a week or two in Aruba . . . without your daughter. This is a situation in which out of sight, out of mind plays a critical role in dealing with the habits and feeding patterns that your toddler has established over the past months. Many mothers find this an easier approach to the withdrawal that toddlers invariably experience when faced with weaning.

Chapter 4

Off to a Solid Start
(Four to Six Months)

Of all the feeding milestones that babies reach during the first few years of life, starting solids has to be one of the most celebrated. What it is about it about the introduction of real food that leads to so much drama and anticipation? Perhaps it represents one of the transitions from baby to little person. Participating in eating means participating in all the social aspects of being a family. Watching a baby experience new textures and flavors gives us something exciting to do, almost as if we're doing it all over again ourselves.

Unfortunately, this excitement can easily turn into anxiety when things don't go just as they're supposed to. What is meant to be a natural transition turns into a stressful transaction between baby and parent. Feeding turns from a fun and rewarding time to a dreaded battle of wills. Part of what initiates this stress effect is the expectations that are put on our babies. These ideas about what a baby is supposed to do are imposed mostly by ourselves as parents but also by family, friends, and marketing executives on Madison Avenue. Our most coveted manuals of child care read like the federal tax code, with more dos and don'ts than a parochial school nun. Baby food manufacturers have created a cottage industry built on pureed vegetables with "stages" of food that always leave us wondering if we're ahead or behind.

Rules are difficult to follow because every baby and every parent is different. Each will offer and take food in a way that is unique to him or her. In her book *Child of Mine— Feeding with Love and Good Sense*, Ellyn Satter relates feeding to a conversation. When we think about good conversation, most of us would agree that both parties have to listen to each other before they can respond in a meaningful way. Successful infant feeding is no different and requires that you listen to your baby and follow her lead. Failure to understand your baby's signals is one of the fundamental problems behind so many difficulties that new parents encounter. Listen to your baby, relax, and enjoy this long-awaited milestone. Don't let rules and regulations interfere with your conversations.

BABY'S FIRST BITES

I'm confused by the term "starting solids." Does this include adding cereal to the bottle?
There's often some misunderstanding when it comes to defining "solids." We typically refer to the initiation of solid feeding as the point at which a baby is fed by spoon. Despite the claims of those fiercely competitive parents who like to think of their babies as advanced, thickening formula unfortunately doesn't qualify.

How do I know my child is ready for solids?
This has to be one of the questions most frequently asked of pediatricians. Despite how monumental an event this seems to be, it's a natural step for babies and one that's easier than most parents anticipate. One of the most important things to remember is that there aren't a whole lot of glaring red flags telling us when a baby's ready to open wide. Other steps in child development are likely to be more obvious. Normal full-term babies are typically ready for solids sometime between four and five months of age. You can talk about rules like "a baby should be able to hold his or her head up" or "she should be able to turn away from food," but most normal four- to six-month-old infants are able to do these things. If, however, you feel compelled to check off a rote list of developmental milestones before picking up the

spoon, go ahead. Just remember that in babies between four and five months, it's most often a leap of faith.

My son was born eight weeks early. Do I start solids at his actual age or corrected age?

For premature infants the rules are a little different because they've been shortchanged time to grow and develop. Keep in mind that your son will be at the growth and developmental equivalent of a normal two-month-old when he reaches four months of age. This is what pediatricians refer to as the *corrected gestational age*. It is established simply by subtracting the number of weeks the baby was born early from his actual age. (Another way to do it is to start counting his age from his due date.) With some exceptions, of course, prematures ultimately catch up by their second birthday, and it's around this time that most pediatricians stop correcting for prematurity.

A former thirty-two-week premature infant is not likely to be ready to jump into solids at four months of age. Wait another month or two until his corrected age is closer to three or four months. This will allow for the development of the skills necessary for safe feeding. The milestones of feeding readiness probably have more application to the former preemie than to full-term babies.

Starting Solids: Ready or Not?

If you have a term baby and you're waiting until at least four or five months to start solids, these signs are probably a moot point since most infants have achieved these milestones by then. If you're looking to start solids earlier than recommended or your baby was a few weeks premature, they're helpful in gauging her readiness for the spoon. She should be able to:

- Hold her head upright and sit with support.
- Lean forward to indicate desire and turn away when not interested in something.
- Show shorter intervals in between feeds and perhaps appear hungry at the end.
- Show some interest in what others are eating around her

Is there any problem with starting solids before four months?
The American Academy of Pediatrics, as well as most pediatricians, recommends waiting until the four-month point before offering that first spoonful of cereal. Despite the fact that some babies are physically capable of eating from a spoon before that time, it is felt that the exposure of the infant bowel to the foreign proteins found in early foods may predispose to food allergy and eczema later.

Four months also marks the time when most important development milestones for feeding are well in place. Most babies are able to support their heads, understand to open their mouths at the sight of a spoon, and indicate satiety by turning away. The *extrusor reflex* also starts to fade around this time. This sometimes frustrating, but important, reflex accounts for the forward thrust of the tongue that is so common of babies when they start solids. Most pediatricians consider the extrusor reflex a natural mechanism to protect babies from having things in their mouths before they're able to safely swallow them. All of these elements together justify the four-month mark as an appropriate, but approximate, age for the initiation of solid food in a baby's diet.

Truth be told, starting your baby on solid food at three and a half months is unlikely to make the sky fall, and if you don't tell your pediatrician he'll never know. Keep in mind, however, that your baby shouldn't need solids earlier than four or even five months of age. Should you feel the urge to pull out the bowl and spoon early, be sure to ask yourself why. Is it to keep at bay an overbearing mother-in-law who insists that the baby's starving? Perhaps you feel the need to keep up with the next-door neighbors who had their baby on three vegetables by six weeks. If your motivations are

---

**Fact or Fiction: Starting Solids Later
Will Help Prevent Obesity Later in Life**

Fiction. There is no solid evidence that early infant feeding practices have any influence on the risk for obesity. Babies do a wonderful job of self-regulating how much and when they need to eat. So let them eat squash!

founded on anything less than sound judgment and patience, remember that there's no rush. Your baby has the rest of his life to eat. A couple of weeks and a little rice cereal won't make any difference in the long run.

Why is rice cereal recommended as the first food to be introduced?

The long-standing recommendation that babies be started on rice cereal is based as much on convention as it is on firm scientific ground. While it may be overrated, there are things about this favored first food that make it a good candidate. Perhaps one of its strongest attributes is its high level of iron. Few starter foods pack as powerful a punch as rice cereal when it comes to iron. This is particularly important for breast-fed infants, where solid foods represent an important source of this critical nutrient.

Rice cereal also contains no gluten. Although it's a controversial issue, it has been suggested that the early introduction of the wheat protein gluten is associated with later onset of gluten enteropathy, or celiac disease. Why rice cereal gets special treatment, however, isn't clear since most of the other first-stage single fruits and vegetables also contain no wheat protein.

Another nice feature about cereals is that they can be mixed to a consistency appropriate to your baby's level of feeding. They can gradually be thickened to provide a more advanced and challenging food source for your baby.

Finally, rice cereal is considered one of the least allergenic first foods. The allergy issue, as usual, is probably overplayed in this case. True immune hypersensitivity to the most common first fruits and vegetables is uncommon enough that it doesn't justify the firm recommendation that rice cereal be first. And if you baby's going to react at four months, he's likely to react at six months.

The bottom line here is that if you start your child with green beans or carrots, the sky is unlikely to fall and your pediatrician (and baby) will never know the difference. But if it gives you a warm, fuzzy feeling to do with your baby what's been done with so many others, by all means go with rice. Just remember that it's an idea backed more by tradition than science.

Is there any difference between *dry* rice cereal and rice cereal out of the jar?

Yes, jarred rice cereal, especially those types containing fruit, contains higher levels of iron than the dry, flaky cereal out of the box. Given the presence of vitamin C found with the fruits, iron absorption may be improved. This difference, however, is probably more trivial than practical. Give your baby what works for her.

Should dry rice cereal be prepared with milk or water?

In most cases this doesn't matter. For the baby who is a poor feeder or who has had difficulty with growth, cereal should be prepared with breast milk or formula in order to maximize calorie intake. For the majority of babies whose intake from the breast or bottle is adequate, water works just fine.

I've heard that dry cereal should be prepared with juice to maximize iron absorption. Is this true?

While the presence of vitamin C from juice may improve the absorption of iron from cereal, the difference shouldn't be significant enough to support its use. In fact, consistently presenting a child's cereal as a sweetened puree may lead to the understanding that all cereal should taste that way. This may set a precedent that's difficult to change once into toddlerhood.

How common is an allergic reaction to rice cereal?

True allergic reactions to rice cereal are exceedingly rare. In fact, allergists in centers dealing with the most unusual and sensitive children with food allergy will tell you that it's almost unheard of. Children will do funny things when they have something new in their system, and rashes occur for many reasons besides food. Don't jump to conclusions after starting on rice and be suspicious of anyone who wants to pin that diagnosis on your child.

Should I offer solids before the bottle or vice versa?
Especially when starting out, give solids before the bottle. If you wait until the end of six ounces of milk, she'll be less motivated to take the spoon when offered. Consider offering the solid portion of her meal first when she's ready to go and follow up with a bottle or breast-feed. Be prepared that a baby's milk intake is typically less after a feed with solids.

In the first few weeks on solids, try not to feed her when she's famished. Doing this may exaggerate the small amount of frustration that's normally felt by babies and parents when starting out.

How much cereal should be given to a baby during the first few days of feeding? How do I know if I've given too much?
When starting out, a baby should receive one to two solid feeds per day. Make sure one is in the morning, since babies (and parents) are more receptive to new things when they're fresh and rested. Initially, feeds should consist of one to two teaspoons of cereal mixed with milk to create a puree with a mushy consistency (about one to two tablespoons of liquid). As a general rule, it should be liquid enough to fall off the spoon if tipped. With time, the amount of food a baby receives should increase.

Knowing when your baby's had enough is something of an art and a skill that you'll need to work on and refine with each stage of feeding development. It's almost impossible to describe, but when a baby's in the middle of a great bowl of cereal or squash, you can almost read her level of satiety by what she's doing. Posture, pace of chewing/smacking, and facial expression all tell a lot. Most babies who are hungry will begin looking for that next spoonful just as soon as they've begun to swallow. As they develop they'll even learn to look into the bowl to see how much is left.

As soon as you begin to see the pace and tempo of the feed begin to wane, it probably means she's reached her capacity. Oftentimes babies will become distracted or fuss more about things that wouldn't have bothered them at the beginning of the feed. At this point you should remark that

The Fear of Feeding

Parents often stress out about feeding. This stress is the consequence of fear, and fear is one of the fundamental emotions driving parents to do the things they do. When I hear exasperated pediatricians talk about "crazy parents," they're usually referring to a mom or dad so overcome with fear that their ability to rationalize and make sound, logical judgment has been disrupted. This is entirely normal and never more evident than when I'm asked to evaluate the child of a pediatrician. It's amazing how even the most experienced, competent pediatrician can lose his or her sense of judgment when dealing with his or her own sick child. No matter how much you know about kids, don't let anyone ever let you believe you're crazy. In most cases your stress and fears are just love and concern gone awry.

So what are the most common fears among parents? If you spend enough time with them, you'll find that a lot of their feeding issues fall under or around one of the following four concerns:

1. I'm going to do something wrong.
There's very little you can do wrong when it comes to feeding your kids. Perhaps the biggest threat to your child is your own fear that things will somehow go awry (or, you have nothing to fear but fear itself). Kids know what to do, and they lack the preoccupations that make parents undermine a healthy feeding relationship. Read the questions found in this book, get the facts, and understand that feeding is natural, not dangerous. There's little you can do to hurt your child in the high chair.

2. My baby is going to have some kind of reaction.
The ever-present fear of a reaction puts some parents in a catatonic state when it comes to feeding. Dangerous reactions to foods are rare, and the most common reactions are temporary and more of a nuisance than a true threat.

3. Something bad will happen if my child doesn't eat.
The parental fixation on the finicky child is almost a cliché. Kids, however, know what they want and how much they want of it. Provide them with limited choices of healthy alternatives and let them do their own thing. When parents interfere with a child's natural drive to regulate her own intake, it leads to feeding struggles that tend to take on a life of their own.

4. My baby is going to choke.
Mothers concerned about choking tend to remain concerned about choking irrespective of what they're told. Choking is thus one of the parental fears most
(continued)

difficult to dispel. If you advance your child on age-appropriate foods with proper supervision, choking shouldn't be an issue. An occasional gag and sputter along the way creates the experiences that collectively allow children to know how to chew and swallow certain foods. This, however, is their issue, not yours. While holding back may seem like the safest thing to do, it's important to understand that the reluctance to advance to age-appropriate foods ultimately can lead to problems like texture aversion.

the next spoonful is the last bite, indicating that feeding time is over. It's important to establish early on the clear expectations about behavior at the end of a feed. While it may seem like a trivial issue at first, establishing such clear boundaries about feeding and its finality is critical to dealing with a toddler.

My mother-in-law insists that our son's baby food be warmed before being given to him. Is this really necessary?
Tactfully tell your mother-in-law that whatever she did in years past doesn't currently apply to your son. It isn't necessary to warm a baby's food, and it's purely personal preference.

How long is baby food good for once a jar is opened?
Refrigerated baby food should be used within forty-eight to seventy-two hours of opening. If in doubt, throw it out. Be sure to feed your child from a bowl and not from the baby food jar. The enzymes and bacteria in your baby's mouth can make their way into the jar and affect the consistency and quality of the food.

I suffered from anorexia nervosa as a teenager and had a great response to therapy. I've been fine since, but I'm worried that this will somehow affect how I feed my daughter. Is this a valid concern?
How eating disorders affect young children is a reasonable concern since these diseases often affect women of childbearing age like yourself. Unfortunately, little substantial

research has been done on the way mothers with eating disorders feed their children. Most of the attention has been paid to the teenage offspring of such mothers since this is when eating disorders tend to appear. What studies have been done show that mothers with eating disorders interact differently with their children when it comes to feeding. Observations have included an absence of positive comments during mealtimes, decreased interaction with their children while feeding, and a tendency to use food for nonnutritive purposes, such as to calm or reward. While it's unclear what relationship these interactions have in *causing* later eating disorders, it seems very likely that they would help set the stage should there be a genetic predisposition for such a disease in a given family.

In your case as an apparently healthy, recovered young

Hyperparenting and the Rush to Advance Solids

In their book *Hyper-Parenting: Are You Hurting Your Child by Trying Too Hard?* Alvin Rosenfeld and Nicole Wise discuss the worrisome trend of pushing our children to their limits. From the compulsive prenatal delivery of classical music to the tight toddler schedules intended to insure maximum development, we have evolved into a society of superachievers.

So too have we become a population of superfeeders. Recent books show us how to "metabolically program" and "fat proof" our children. The "next-generation" diet is pushed by a physician expert whose claim to fame is that he himself was obese as a child. The list goes on as the market tries to quench our thirst for quick fixes and catchy methods to make our children nutritional superachievers.

This drive to push children nutritionally is first seen with the introduction of solid food. Many parents seem to be obsessed with the early initiation of solids. Whether it's the myth of nighttime solitude or the competitive nature of some parents to want to boast about the accelerated skills of their baby, many parents push hard to get their babies to take this step. Be aware that forcing a baby to do something before she's prepared can have consequences that will follow her through childhood. Dysfunctional feeding is often a consequence of forcing something that isn't quite ready to fit. Whether it's your competitive nature or pressure from family and friends, don't let hyperparenting find its way to your baby's high chair.

woman with a history of an eating disorder, your awareness is your best defense. Understanding the potential for problems is the first means of preventing them. Read this book, understand the basics of how to handle different situations, and look for help if you have concerns.

BEYOND RICE

Does a baby have to take every single grain cereal before advancing to fruits or vegetables?

Some parents have the idea that their baby can't eat anything more advanced until she's tried every grain available in the grocery store. If you're one of them, you need to reconsider your source of information. If you've chosen to start your baby on rice cereal, you can feel free to start fruits or vegetables at any time. There's no need to cover every grain before moving on. Remember too that there's no law (that I'm aware of) dictating that babies be started on cereals. Fruits and vegetables make fine first foods.

Is there a critical order of introduction for foods?

No. In fact, there's nothing at all in the feeding process that should be looked on as critical. Feeding your baby should be a relaxed, enjoyable experience, and it's very, very hard for anyone to get hurt. The only consideration to keep in mind is

---

Grandmothers and Feeding—No Fear

While you may think Grandma's pushy and full of old-fashioned ideas, keep in mind that she's actually done this before. If you've never noticed, grandmothers have an instinctive let's-go-for-it attitude when it comes to feeding. They're constantly pushing the limits of what babies should do with their mouths. Why is this true? Because they aren't inhibited by any of the four fundamental fears of feeding kids. They've done it before and they know that there aren't too many places to drop the ball. While I can't agree with the nearly universal drive by grandmothers to push solids before their time, I think there's something to be said for the reassuring confidence that Grandma brings to the high chair.

The Feeding Police

You may recall that when you were pregnant there was never a shortage of people to tell you what to do, what to eat, and what not to eat. You lived through the horror stories of what would happen to your unborn baby if you took a sip of a diet cola or thought about a glass of wine. Unfortunately, these well-intentioned and seemingly all-knowing people who followed you through your pregnancy don't disappear after your baby is born. They're referred to as the feeding police, and they're one of the motivating factors behind this book.

Who are they? The feeding police comprise a large underground of individuals whose goal is to undermine your confidence as a parent. They frequently patrol play groups, playgrounds, pediatricians' waiting rooms, and anyplace frequented by young, inexperienced parents.

How can I tell if I'm dealing with them? In general, they have a way of making you feel as if you're apt to do irreparable damage to your baby if you don't listen to them. *Other characteristics include*:

- Offering advice when it isn't requested
- Thinking they know everything
- Having an answer to every question
- Having a source of information (pediatrician, latest book or article) that they claim is the ultimate and final source of reference.

What can I do?

- First understand that they have no authority over the way you raise or feed your child.
- Don't hate them. The majority have underlying personality issues that lead them into this self-imposed position of authority.
- Understand that solid information is your best defense. If there are questions, report them to your pediatrician and get the facts.

---

that single foods should be introduced one at a time in order to identify any type of intolerance or allergy. You can introduce new foods as early as four days after a previous food has been introduced.

Note: As you'll figure out, the order of introduction of foods is prime fodder for the feeding police. And it's amazing the range of opinions that exist about how to offer a baby a bowl of squash. But don't let 'em break your stride. If you find yourself deliberating over which comes first, sweet potatoes or green beans, ask yourself one question: Will this matter twenty years from now?

What's the difference between first-, second-, and third-stage foods?

Some parents place a lot of stock in the stage of food that their baby is on. The staging of foods by manufacturers is a fairly arbitrary system of grading a food's consistency or lumpiness. Stage 1 is effectively liquidy pureed food and stage 3 is pureed food with moderately large residual lumps of solid food. Stage 2 is closer in consistency to stage 1 foods but is often sold in larger jars to meet the appetite of more advanced infants. There are no strict rules or age guidelines for the advancement of a baby's food texture. Babies, of course, should be started on pureed foods between four and six months of age. More advanced textured foods (stage 3) can and should be offered around seven or eight months of age. Some children will transition to squashed table food before reaching stage 3 foods.

How do I know when it's OK to switch from stage 1 to stage 2 foods?

This is something that requires neither a license nor permission from your pediatrician. The difference between most stage 1 and stage 2 foods is *size of the jar* and the availability of a more diverse *combination of foods*. The texture shouldn't be any more advanced than that found in stage 1 foods. So if your child is polishing away his stage 1s and takes a small variety of fruits and vegetables (four to six), feel free to take the leap. Just be aware of the addition of

---

Fact or Fiction: Starting Fruits Before Vegetables Will Lead a Baby to Prefer Sweets and Dislike Vegetables

Fiction. There's no evidence that the order of introduction of different foods has any influence on the outcome of taste preference. Start with whatever you like. If the feeding police threaten you, refer them to this book.

new fruits, veggies, or other foods that may not have been present in any of her individual stage 1 servings. This is important in the event of an allergic reaction.

What bowel changes can we expect as our baby makes the transition to solids?

Parents love to count, measure, describe, and document what does or doesn't appear inside their baby's diaper. What makes this fascination so universal among parents isn't entirely clear except that it seems to be fueled by the addition of solids to the diet.

So what is it about solids that'll change the way you see a dirty diaper? When you begin your baby on food, you're introducing a whole new variety of nutritional substrates to her digestive system. The new sugars found in fruits and vegetables will change the amount and types of bacteria in the colon. The fat composition of a solid diet will change the speed at which things move through the intestine. And on top of these radical dietary changes, your baby's bowel is growing and maturing. As one would expect, all of these transitions add up to an altogether different-looking stool. While this may seem alarming, it's entirely normal.

Look for the following changes in your baby's diaper as you begin solids:

- *Frequency*. In general, feeding shouldn't have a dramatic impact on how frequently he poops. A baby's stooling pattern can change temporarily while something new is in the system, but this typically passes within a few days.
- *Odor*. Stool gets its foul odor from the bacteria that live and grow in the colon. The bacteria that inhabit the colon and make up the bulk of a baby's stool are influenced by the food in his diet. As new sugars make their way into the colon, different types of bacteria grow and prosper. The result can be stinky poop.
- *Color*. Unless you're picking avocados or looking for shoes to match your bag, color really doesn't matter. Your baby's stool can appear to have funny colors de-

pending on what's eaten and how it is digested. And with very few exceptions, it's of no significance. Remember that as your baby moves beyond pureed vegetables it's not uncommon to see UVOs (unidentified vegetable objects) passing through into the diaper.

- *Consistency.* Almost universally, a baby's stool consistency will change with solids. This can run the gamut from firm and difficult to pass to loose and slimy. Of all the changes you'll observe in your baby's stool, consistency is likely to be the only one that you'll need to act on. Loose, runny bowel movements that develop with the addition of a new food can mean any number of problems. For most babies this means simply that she isn't quite prepared yet to deal with that particular food (simple intolerance). It may indicate an allergic reaction, although in the absence of rash or vomiting, this can be difficult to prove. Be careful about permanently writing off a certain food because of a "reaction" or unusual-looking stool. If your child has a runny diaper with bananas, try again in a couple of months when her digestive system is a little better adjusted.
- Firm stools that require straining are common with any of the cereals, and you may need to limit these. While cereals are a terrific source of iron, babies can live without them.

When should a child begin taking three solid feeds a day?

As discussed, when you start your baby on solid food, you typically will offer food twice a day. As soon as a baby is used to the concept of solids, it's reasonable to transition him to three meals a day just like the rest of the family. An appropriate time to make this transition is around seven months.

The move to three feeds a day is an exciting milestone because it signals that your baby is starting to eat like other members of the family. Assuming that you eat together as a family at least once or twice a day, this social pattern of feeding is extremely important because it enables the baby or toddler to learn what is expected of them.

Family meals should encourage and reinforce the following mealtime rules:

- Meals are eaten at reasonably set times.
- Meals have a beginning and an end.
- Sometimes it's necessary to be patient and wait to eat even though we may be hungry.
- While we may choose how much we want to eat at any given meal, we all have to choose our foods from what's presented to us.
- Eating is as much a social experience as it is a biological need.
- Certain behaviors are acceptable and others unacceptable at the table.

When is it OK to introduce meats?
Meat can be introduced anytime after seven months of age. While babies don't necessarily need meat, it offers a terrific source of iron. It becomes even more important when you consider that the intake of iron-rich cereal decreases later in the first year to be replaced by more interesting fruit and vegetable combinations. And not all iron is created equal. The type of iron found in meat is absorbed more efficiently than that found in cereals or fortified foods. So despite the fact that infants can get by without meat, don't be cavalier about brushing aside this rich source of iron.

I've noticed that some baby foods contain starch fillers. Are these safe for babies?
Starches are a natural type of carbohydrate that may be added to food in the form of flour (corn, wheat, rice), tapioca, or rice. Starches are added to food to control its texture and consistency. They are safe for infants, and the FDA requires that they be listed on food labels.

I've heard that traditional baby food can contain traces of pesticide from the vegetables used in their ingredients. Is this true and is it enough to consider trying organic baby food?

Despite the pure image that our favorite baby food manufacturers convey, studies by both the FDA and independent labs have demonstrated the presence of pesticide residue in jarred baby food. While we may find comfort in the fact that the levels of pesticide contamination fall well below what federal standards consider safe, it's unclear how much is too much. This is especially true when it comes to children since the toxicological significance of early exposure to these residues is not known.

Whether you consider this a cause for serious concern depends on how you look at things. If you see exposure to environmental toxins as an inevitable consequence of being a passenger on the planet, the traces found in baby food are unlikely to faze you. If, however, you find that the uncertain significance of this kind of exposure to your baby leaves you sleepless, look elsewhere for your baby's food. The cost to your sanity is worth the effort to find or make food that you at least think is clean.

Judging Baby Food by Its Cover

What you see on a baby food label may tell you a lot about what's inside:

- *Order of ingredients*. Manufacturers are required to disclose the relative quantities of the ingredients in their foods by listing the most abundant ingredient first.
- *Water*. Water often is added to pureed vegetables during manufacturing. While you may think that this would dilute the nutritional quality of the food, it's rarely enough to be significant.
- *Starch and other additives*. Starches often are added to provide texture to baby food. Watch for the addition of salt and sugar, since these shouldn't be part of your child's diet at this age.
- *Fortified with* . . . This describes the addition of important nutrients and minerals to ensure that babies get what they need. An example is iron in cereal.
- Natural and not-so-natural. Be careful about the ingredients described as "natural." By definition, ingredients such as salt and corn syrup are considered natural. Food described as "organic" is probably a good thing, although there are new standards in place for organic labeling. Be sure you know what you're buying.

As a possible solution to this whole dilemma, some manufacturers recently have begun offering organically prepared selections of baby food. By most standards, organically grown food is food grown and processed using no synthetic fertilizers or pesticides. The U.S. Department of Agriculture has recently released new national standards for the production, handling, and processing of organically grown food that require labeling depending upon how much of the food's content is truly organic. And how organic any baby food manufacturer chooses to make their food has yet to be determined. Use of the new organic labeling standards is currently under way with full implementation by manufacturers expected by the summer of 2002. Helping you decide how organic you want your child's food is well beyond the scope of this book, however. Ultimately you'll need to take a leap of faith and understand that the stress generated by your concern is potentially as dangerous as what's on the end of the spoon.

Is homemade baby food more nutritious than jarred baby food?

The word "nutritious" can mean any number of things, depending on your point of view or what you're accustomed to eating. While it can be argued that vacuum-sealed jarred vegetables may have subtle nutritional differences when compared with kitchen-prepared, freezer-stored vegetables, the differences aren't significant enough to warrant turning your kitchen upside down. For many parents the fresh nature of what they prepare on their own, the absence of additives or fillers, and the hands-on love that is part of their food preparation make homemade baby food more worthwhile.

Don't Try This at Home

If you choose to prepare your own baby food, be sure to avoid beets, turnips, carrots, and collard greens for the first year. These vegetables contain natural compounds called *nitrates* that, when taken in excess, can interfere with the way red blood cells carry oxygen. Unfortunately, you can't test for nitrates yourself so it's best off to avoid them altogether in your homemade baby food. Baby food manufacturers are aware of this issue and monitor their products for safe levels of nitrates.

Providing your child with a menu of safe, properly prepared first foods requires a little education, some attention to detail, and a commitment of time. Since the art and science of baby food preparation is beyond the scope of this book, look for Ruth Yaron's *Super Baby Food*. It represents an excellent primer on the safe preparation and storage of home-made baby food.

SOLID STRUGGLES

We recently introduced cereal to our four-and-a-half-month-old, and whatever goes in her mouth comes right back out. Is this normal?

Yes, this is entirely normal, and it doesn't mean she isn't ready for solids. This natural reaction to "tongue" out anything that feels funny is referred to as the *extrusor reflex*. All babies have this natural protective mechanism, and it's what keeps babies from trying to swallow things that they're not yet ready to have. Unfortunately, despite how mature or ready a baby is to feed, the first several days are often met with what some parents feel is rejection of solids. Assuming that you haven't started solids too early (around four months for a term baby), this transient and short-lived reflex should be handled with gentle persistence. Continue to offer one to two solid feeds daily with each feed consisting of four to five spoons (or attempted spoons).

Note: Some parenting manuals note that one of the signs of readiness for solids is the ability of a baby to keep food in her mouth. This is absolutely absurd. If some persistence of the extrusor reflex weren't normal, we wouldn't have bibs, and if we followed this rule, no baby would ever be allowed to eat.

My five-and-a-half-month-old refuses to eat cereal. He has done beautifully with the fruits we have offered but continues to refuse cereal. Is this OK?

This is OK. The reason that cereals are preferred as the first food is that they are believed to be the least allergenic of the first foods offered to infants. Despite this fact, the incidence of true allergic reactions to the basic fruits and vegetables offered to babies is also quite low.

Another reason that cereal is one of the favored infant foods is that it is represents a terrific source of iron—a frequent nutritional sore spot in the first year of life. A baby's diet at this age is typically rich in fruits and vegetables and often lacks any significant source of iron. This becomes less of an issue later in the first year, when the diet comes to include foods like meat.

With that said, skipping cereal shouldn't present a major problem for your baby. If bottle-feeding, provide your baby with an iron-supplemented formula. If you are breast-feeding, an iron supplement would be recommended starting at about six months. Finally, you might want to consider alternative ways of getting your baby to take cereal. Try buying mixed cereal-fruit combinations or mixing her favorite fruit with cereal in a proportion she finds acceptable.

Gagging

All babies will gag from time to time and while you may look upon it as a life-threatening event, it's really a sophisticated safeguard. Gagging is a protective mechanism that keeps food from passing into the windpipe where it doesn't belong. Should your baby attempt to talk while eating and begin to take a breath full of food, the muscles of the pharynx will force that food back where it came from. While it may appear dramatic, the effects of a lungful of green beans are far more impressive.

Some gagging is acceptable from time to time at this age. It's part of the process of learning how to manipulate and swallow foods of different size and texture. It should be an infrequent event, however. If you notice that your baby gags frequently with solids, she should be evaluated by your physician. While this most likely represents a minor developmental speed bump, it may require further tests.

If gagging is the protective reflex, choking is what that reflex is trying to prevent. Choking is what occurs when food actually makes its way into the airway. The hallmark of the choking child is the silent absence of noise and airflow. Since air can neither move in or out, the child often appears frozen and terrified. As opposed to so many of the things that parents get excited about, this truly constitutes an emergency.

Is it possible for a five-month-old not to like a certain food?
Absolutely. While it may not be carried out with the style
and flair of a toddler, a baby clearly has the ability to discern
tastes at this age. And as soon as a baby can close her mouth,
turn away, pull back, or put on a sour face, she can display
these preferences. Such preferences aren't anything to get
too excited about, however. Most are short-lived and rarely
evolve into any long-standing pattern of tastes. The source
of today's sour face is tomorrow's obsession.

At what age are babies able to detect saltiness in food?
While the amazing newborn palate appears to be able to discriminate the sensations of sweet, sour, and bitter, the idea
of saltiness is appreciated only after about four months of
age. But don't get any ideas. The salt shaker should have no
role in the feeding of any infant. And while it may seem like
a good short-term solution for the finicky first feeder, studies
show that, over the long term, babies consume salted foods
no better than unsalted foods.

How long should a hunger strike from teething last?
While it may sound evasive, it depends on the baby. For
most, the temporary rejection of solids lasts no more than a
couple of days at this age. Once a baby achieves the level of
modified table food and starts to erupt a molar or two, this
strike can last a week or more.

GUT REACTIONS—FOOD ALLERGY AND INTOLERANCE

How long should we wait when introducing new foods?
You should keep your baby on a new food as long as it takes
to make absolutely sure you're not going to see an allergic
reaction. While I consider a week the optimal time to test-
drive a food, you're probably OK if your child goes three to
five days with no reaction. If you're watching the big hand
on the clock to know when your five days are up, you're trying to go too fast. Remember that besides trying to keep up

---

Medically Speaking: Allergy vs. Intolerance

Purists often "react" when they hear these two words mixed up.

Intolerance describes any unusual or undesirable symptom that occurs from a food. An example is the gas, bloating, and cramping that occurs in some people after ingesting the milk sugar lactose. An otherwise healthy baby who has loose stools after eating green beans may be considered "intolerant" of green beans. Food intolerance can produce symptoms very similar to an allergic response, but they do not involve the immune system.

Allergy is a very specific type of reaction that involves an *immune response* to a protein in the diet. An immune response is a very specific physiologic process the body uses to defend itself against foreign proteins. It can involve the recruitment of white blood cells and the production of antibodies, or specific proteins that help fight infection. An example would be the hives and wheezing that some children experience with peanuts. While a very bad allergic reaction may be recognizable based on a child's signs and symptoms, blood and skin testing may be necessary in some cases.

---

with other kids in the neighborhood, there's no reason to rush your baby into a varied and complex diet. She has all of her life to experience the variety of different foods, and at this age she should be happy with just about anything.

What foods are most likely to cause allergy?
Fortunately, the fruits and vegetables that babies start with during their first few months of feeding infrequently cause true allergic reactions. And a preoccupation with allergic reactions shouldn't be part of your feeding experience as a parent. Feeding should be a relaxed and enjoyable time and shouldn't involve the fear and anticipation that comes with defusing a bomb. Even if your baby does experience an allergic reaction, it's unlikely to be as dramatic as anything seen on *Mission: Impossible*.

The most common allergies experienced by children are to milk, wheat, egg, fish, and peanut. Most milk allergies in infants are picked up in the first few months of life through the use of standard formula or breast milk. Peanut exposure through crushed nuts, butter, or oils should certainly be avoided during the first year. (The nuts themselves, should be considered a choking hazard until a child is at least four years old.) Wheat protein should be withheld until after eight months.

Keep in mind that these perpetrators may be hidden in table foods and mixed baby foods. It may take some detective work (and the help of an allergist) to identify the culprit should your baby have a significant reaction.

My son was diagnosed with milk allergy at four weeks of age and has been fed with Nutramigen (casein hydrolysate formula). He's five months old now, and we would like to start him on solids. We're nervous about it. Is there anything we need to look for?
This is a very common concern among parents of children with milk protein hypersensitivity. The fear is that if he's allergic to milk protein, he'll also be at risk for a number of other allergies. As it turns out, most babies with milk reactivity as infants do just fine advancing on solids as any other baby would. We typically recommend that babies such as your son start with cereals at four months of age with no particular precautions.

The baby with *severe* protein hypersensitivity who has exhibited signs of significant bleeding, rash, or breathing difficulties should be treated differently, however. While most of the infants in this category will advance to baby foods without a problem, the more sensitive infants are at risk for reacting to certain baby food components, such as soy protein. If you believe your son fits into the category of severe protein reactivity,

Signs of Food Allergy

The most common symptoms of food allergy in children are hives, rash, wheezing, congestion, diarrhea, vomiting, and cramping. At this age most of these symptoms should be seen within a few hours of exposure to the food in question. Unfortunately, the signs that typically indicate allergy can appear for a variety of other reasons. Congestion, for example, is frequently reported by new parents, and it can indicate any number of problems, including upper respiratory infection, reflux, and environmental allergy. While you should watch for these symptoms, be cautious about self-diagnosing allergy when only one of them is present.

discuss his case with an experienced pediatric gastroenterologist before advancing to solids.

Why is it recommended that wheat be withheld until seven or eight months?

While controversial, there's some evidence to support the idea that early exposure to wheat is associated with the later onset of celiac disease. Celiac disease is a condition in which the lining of the intestine reacts to a particular protein found in wheat. Children with celiac disease typically suffer from chronic diarrhea and malnutrition due to malabsorption of nutrients.

How early exposure to food is related to this disease requires a little understanding of the baby intestine. Early in life the lining of the intestine is leaky and readily allows foreign protein to get into the bloodstream. What this means is that the small segments of protein that comprise a baby's food can get into the bloodstream and initiate the production of antibodies. Antibodies are the components of our immune system responsible for identifying and targeting foreign proteins. As long as these antibodies are present (most of our lives), the body is programmed to react should it ever encounter that particular protein again. These reactions are what we typically associate with allergy.

So it seems that offering a baby foreign proteins such as wheat before the bowel is mature may allow the immune system to get programmed and play a role in the later development of celiac disease. But wheat normally doesn't play much of a role in the diet of most infants fed a typical Western baby diet. In addition to wheat, the protein responsible for this condition can be found in barley, rye, and possibly oats. This does not mean that you shouldn't offer your baby barley or oats. As with all diseases, their development requires a genetic predisposition in addition to environmental exposures. If you have a strong family history of celiac disease, these cereals probably should be avoided until late in the first year, although rice is still fine.

Whether your baby is at risk or not, this issue reinforces

Fact or Fiction: The Foods You Eat While Pregnant Could Set Your Child Up for Later Allergies

Fiction. While a long-standing suspicion among those who treat food allergy, there is no convincing evidence that in utero exposure to food protein predisposes to problems after birth.

---

the idea of advancing babies at a slow pace. There's no advantage to pushing your baby, and, as in this case, there may be potential risks.

When is it safe to start a baby on eggs?

Despite the fact that eggs make a terrific food for self-feeding babies, they probably should be withheld until twelve months of age. If there is a strong family history of allergy to egg, twenty-four months would be a safer starting point. Egg yolks, which are less allergenic, can be introduced as early as eight months. Eggs served scrambled or hard-boiled make good finger foods for young toddlers.

Are egg substitutes safe for children who are allergic to eggs?

Absolutely not. Egg substitutes exist primarily for fat and cholesterol issues and unfortunately contain egg protein. They are unsafe for individuals with known or suspected egg allergy.

Food Allergy on the Net

Be careful where you go and what you listen to, especially when it comes to food allergy. If you want reliable information without the hype, check out *www.foodallergy.org*. Maintained by the Food Allergy Network, an organization dedicated to public education on allergy, this is a fantastic resource for parents of children with significant food allergy. Most important, some of the country's preeminent allergists serve on its advisory board and regularly contribute to its content.

Chapter 5

Solid Transitions
(Six to Twelve Months)

As in all aspects of raising children, once you answer one question, another one comes along to get you thinking. It seems just as soon as you answer "What foods should we start with?" you're asking "What shouldn't he be eating?" It never ends. Despite the new questions, late infancy will bring your infant further from pureed baby food and closer to the table. He will move from two feeds a day to three and begin to eat with and like the rest of the family.

Along with the novelty of more advanced foods comes the issues of feeding refusal and other behavioral problems that are nothing more than a foreshadowing of toddlerhood. Feeding starts to transcend a biological process whereby the baby takes the fuel he needs and evolves to become part of an emotional, social process that can be either rewarding or frustrating, depending on the day.

ADVANCED SOLIDS

My baby eats a lot of squash and carrots and I have noticed that her skin is a slight shade of yellow. Is this jaundice?
This is a condition referred to as carotenemia, and it results from the excessive intake of a pigment called carotene. Carotene is abundant in orange and yellow vegetables, and your child's slight skin discoloration reflects her appeal for these vegetables. It's absolutely harmless and will fade with the addition of other foods to her diet.

Jaundice is a condition in which the level of bilirubin in the blood elevates due to a variety of medical conditions.

Bilirubin is a normal by-product of liver metabolism and is released into the intestines, where it plays a role in fat absorption and gives stool its golden hue. One of the ways you can distinguish carotenemia from jaundice is that in children with jaundice, the whites of the eyes are also yellow. Carotenemia doesn't involve the eyes.

My son is seven months old and we haven't yet offered him solids. Is there any danger in waiting to introduce solids?

While the word "danger" may be a bit strong, it wouldn't be a good idea to keep your child away from solids much longer. After six months of age, children enter a critical period where they learn to accept the new textures and sensations that solids provide. The introduction of these new sensations can be delayed until seven or eight months, but pushing things much beyond that risks the development of what's referred to as an oral aversion. If there ever was a danger in delaying solids, this is it.

The term "oral aversion" refers to a hypersensitivity to normal oral stimulation. It can be thought of as an anxiety-based response to something that the child either is afraid of or isn't willing to accept. It can occur when a child is fearful of certain textures that he has never encountered. This is often the case with the child who is never introduced to solids until late in the first year. Oral aversion also can occur when a child learns to associate a particular oral stimulus with some painful event such as swallowing. Babies with recurrent heartburn, or reflux, often learn to avoid solids because of fear of pain.

While I normally don't push parents to start their children on food until they feel comfortable, the potential for aversion illustrates the importance of getting things under way by at least six months of age, even if only in small amounts. We take for granted what a huge step it is for an infant to process the sensory information that goes along with starting solids. And unfortunately, this is a step that isn't fully appreciated until we see a child in whom the introduction of solids has been delayed significantly.

Medically Speaking: Oral Aversion

Definition: Negative response to oral stimulation that occurs when a child is faced with a taste or texture that he or she either isn't accustomed to or has previously associated with pain.

Symptoms: The most common sign of oral aversion is choking or gagging with solid textures. Some children will react to any oral stimulation, including use of a spoon or even touching around the mouth.

Cause: Most often the result of late introduction of solids, a negative feeding experience, or some history of painful swallowing (reflux).

Treatment: Typically requires oral motor therapy prescribed by a physician and provided by a pediatric occupational therapist or speech therapist. This consists of deconditioning exercises (with and without food) aimed at getting the child to accept various forms of oral stimulation. Treatment can take weeks to months.

How much cereal does my baby need after six months to give him the iron he needs?

While there is nothing magical about cereal, it does provide a valuable source of iron for babies during the last six months of their first year. How much cereal a baby needs to meet her iron needs depends entirely on her intake of formula or breast milk. Children at this age need approximately 10 milligrams of iron per day, which should be met with twenty-seven ounces of regular infant formula. If, for some reason, you have chosen to provide your baby with low-iron formula, she would need to consume *eighty-three ounces a day* to meet her iron needs. This is, of course, impossible and illustrates why low-iron formulas should have no role in any child's diet.

So assuming that you're providing your child with regular infant formula, her need for cereal or other iron-containing food will depend on whether she's meeting all of her needs with formula. Typically a baby's intake of formula will fall under the twenty-seven-ounce mark once solids begin to pick up speed later in the first year. How much cereal or other iron-containing food your child requires will depend on how much formula she's actually taking. Since you should never use a calculator when feeding your baby, don't get caught up in counting milligrams of iron. Instead, encourage intake of *at least* a half-ounce, or four tablespoons, a day of dry cereal with formula or cereal with fruit. This should provide approximately half of your child's daily need for iron with the remainder being made up with formula and other foods. After seven or eight months the introduction of meats will make your cereal compulsion less of an issue.

My child is nine months old and eats a variety of foods. Does he still need to get cereal?

Assuming that your child takes in appropriate quantities of breast milk or iron-supplemented formula in addition to iron-rich foods like meat, cereal will become less important later in the first year. Considering that meats may not make it onto the high chair on a daily basis, be sure to offer a serving of cereal or cereal with fruit during at least one meal a day. Usually at this age children are beginning to look beyond the high chair to what's being served to the rest of the family. Look at this interest in table food as an opportunity to expand her diet and provide some alternative sources of iron, such as

> **Three Times as Big**
>
> Your baby's birth weight should triple at around a year of age.

wheat germ, egg noodles, beans, peas, and different types of bread.

How do I know my baby's ready for table food?

At the risk of sounding picky, it all depends on how you define table food. To some this is food in the form that we would eat it as adults; to others, table food is anything that doesn't come from a baby food jar. For the sake of this book, we'll consider table food as something that we as adults may eat but perhaps in a form that's safe and acceptable for a baby or toddler.

Unfortunately, babies don't offer a lot of obvious clues about table-food readiness. Beginning around eight months

---

Fact or Fiction: Babies Need Teeth Before Taking Table Food

Fiction. When it comes to advancing babies on solid food, teeth are highly over-rated. Modified adult foods or table food can be offered to babies as early as eight months of age. At this age, and for the months to come, a baby's dental pattern consists primarily of incisors, or biting teeth. While the incisors may help a child cut a generous piece of melon in two, they have a minor role in getting food prepared for swallowing. The molars, which are involved with chewing and grinding, aren't involved in a child's eating until partway into the second year.

---

of age, most babies will begin to take interest in what's beyond the confines of their high chair. This interest may be limited to nothing more than a curiosity about the colors and shapes on your plate. Some babies, however, will actually begin to refuse their silky-textured baby food—a sign that they're ready for something more advanced.

If your baby is at least eight months old and you suspect that she may be growing tired of the same old dull routine, try offering some mashed baked potato or squash from your plate (unseasoned, of course). If it seems to arouse a new attitude in your fickle feeder, you may be on to something.

How does a baby's formula or breast milk intake change as solids are advanced?

As might be expected, a baby's milk intake should decrease as her intake of solids picks up. In fact, a baby's daily milk volume peaks at approximately four to six months of age at thirty to thirty-eight ounces per day. Milk intake decreases progressively to approximately twenty to twenty-eight ounces per day at twelve months of age.

Parents frequently are concerned that this drop in milk intake will cause a baby to fall short in the calories important for growth and development. While it's true that the replacement of a baby's fatty, protein-rich milk with low-calorie fruits and vegetable results in a transient dip in caloric intake, this is more than compensated for by the addition of meats and complex foods later in the first year.

How much formula should a nine-month-old be taking? My son takes three six-ounce bottles per day in addition to three hearty meals of baby and table food. I'm concerned that this isn't enough.

Anyone who spends enough time with kids knows that firm rules of intake are rarely applicable to real life. With that said, most babies between the ages of six and nine months will take anywhere from twenty-five to thirty-five ounces of formula in a day. This depends on how often a bottle is offered, who's caring for the child, the availability of other liquids, and how interested the baby is in solids. At a year this will drop to about twenty to twenty-eight ounces in a day with the average being about twenty-two ounces.

In the case of your child, eighteen ounces a day in addition to what appears to be a healthy solid appetite is a little less than what the average child this age takes. This shouldn't be cause for concern, however, since plenty of healthy, thriving babies get by on this amount of formula. Be sure that you're not offering juice or sports drinks instead of milk since breast milk or formula should be the preferred beverage during the first year. Water is a reasonable supplement but shouldn't be required in amounts over four to six ounces a day.

When Is a Baby Fattest?

A baby's body reaches its greatest percentage of fat at approximately nine months of age.

Finally, growth should be the bottom line when talking about the adequacy of a child's diet. Regular visits to your pediatrician during the first year should involve close monitoring of your child's growth.

My eleven-month-old has always been a great feeder, but recently she has begun refusing baby food. What should I do?

While feeding refusal can represent any number of problems, your daughter's fickle behavior is probably entirely normal. This behavior, while frustrating, is appropriate and represents her curiosity and willingness to perhaps imitate the way you feed yourself. If you haven't done so already, this may be the time to offer soft, mushy table food such as

---

It's Never Too Early to Bring Your Baby to the Table

As inconvenient as it may seem, be sure to make time for meals together. Early on children learn through example the rules and regulations of mealtime behavior. And the benefits of eating together go beyond behavior and actually encourage good nutrition. A recent study has shown that children from families that eat together are more likely to take the recommended five servings a day of fruits and vegetables. In addition, family meals have been associated with improved vocabulary and better self-esteem in children. Even if it's just once a day, start a healthy family routine and bring your baby to the table.

---

mashed potatoes, squash, squashed banana, or oatmeal. At this age a baby also should be on a fairly regular schedule of three meals per day with two snacks. Eating with the rest of the family will help establish the pattern that she's just like everyone else and ultimately should be expected to eat like everyone else. (This is, of course, assuming that your family sits down on some regular basis to eat together. Remember, good habits start early.)

If you notice that your daughter isn't interested in table food and continues to refuse her baby food, have her evaluated by your pediatrician since her problem could represent a treatable condition like oral thrush or an ear infection.

I understand that children aren't supposed to drink regular milk until a year or so. Can cooked table foods be prepared with whole milk?
Yes, the table foods that babies take in late infancy may contain whole milk. The amount found in these foods is not enough to cause the harm that we typically associate with milk use in infants.

Is it OK to give yogurt to a baby before a year of age?
Despite the fact that yogurt would seem to be the ideal first food, it does contain cow's milk protein. But like other milk-containing table foods that babies get into late in their first year, the quantities are usually limited and we tend not to get too concerned over this degree of milk exposure. To avoid any potential problem, yogurt should probably be re-

served for after eight months with daily quantities limited to two to four ounces per day. Stick with the plain, nonsweetened variety and add your own soft, minced fruit to keep things interesting. Yogurt should be withheld from babies who have a documented milk protein allergy and introduced only under the direction of your pediatrician.

How early can children begin to drink juice?

It should be understood that no child of any age needs juice. While we tend to think of juices as a valuable source of vitamins and minerals, most babies get those vitamins and minerals through a well-balanced diet including milk and solids. It's probably safe to offer juice as early as six months of age, although a good goal might be to wait until she's drinking from a tippy cup. This may create a novel incentive for transition to an alternative way of drinking. Juice should be limited to approximately four to five ounces a day and should be seen as a way to provide variety and additional fluid to her diet.

Is there any difference between regular juice and the juice sold by baby food manufacturers?

Juice is juice no matter how you package it. While baby food manufacturers appropriately sell 100% juice fortified with vitamins, it shouldn't be any different from any other juice. If you prefer a teddy bear or a smiling baby adorning the label of your child's juice, be prepared to pay a premium, however. Infant juices tend to be more expensive per ounce than many "adult" juices.

SELF-SERVING BABIES

When should a child begin self-feeding?

Most children will begin to show an interest in feeding themselves around nine or ten months of age. It's around this time that you can begin preparing small portions of soft, diced food, such as well-cooked vegetables, diced fruit, or

Cheerios. Remember that self-feeding doesn't mark the end of the bowl and spoon! Your baby will still need the nutritional variety that comes from baby food and mashed table food.

Form Follows Function

Babies typically develop a *superior pincer grasp* at nine to ten months, which is one of the reasons finger foods are such a hit. Not only do small pieces of diced food provide a new and funky feeding experience for the child, it allows them to exercise their newfound fine motor skills!

How early can I begin offering zwieback toast or teething biscuits to my child?

While most teething biscuits are designed to become soft and melt away on chewing, larger pieces can break off and present a choking hazard to a child. Because of this remote but possible risk, teething biscuits should be introduced to your baby at ten to twelve months of age and then only under close supervision. If he's more interested in using his jaw to break the biscuit into pieces, it may not be such a good idea. Consider instead the use of unsalted saltines, which have a melt-away quality and present much less of risk for choking.

Fabulous Finger Foods

- Cooked veggies like carrot spears, potatoes, avocados, green beans, broccoli trees
- Fruit such as banana slices, ripe melon, ripe pear slices, diced peaches
- Well-cooked pasta such as fusilli or elbow macaroni
- Small pancakes
- Cheerios
- Graham crackers

Our baby spends more time smearing his food on the high chair or on his face. What can I do to get him more interested in putting it in his mouth?

This is terrific! Nothing helps get a child better acquainted with the texture of his food than feeling it on his skin and in his hair. Remember that feeding is a multisensory experience, and compulsive cleanliness can lead to problems accepting different kinds of food and enjoying mealtime. If you have a problem with your son using sweet potatoes as hair gel, grab the camera and remember: If he's hungry he'll find his mouth.

Finger (Feeding) Tips

- **Don't put out too much.** Limit the selection to two or three pieces at one time. This will prevent overstuffing and overstimulation. Too much selection can lead to frustration.
- **Make sure it's small.** It should be small enough that she won't choke on it if she swallows it whole. A good gauge is that food pieces should be smaller than the width of her pinkie.
- **Offer the spoon feeding first.** Once your child experiences the novelty of self-feeding, you may find her resistant to the traditional bowl and spoon. If non–finger foods are on the menu, offer these before the more colorful and enticing fruit chunks are spread before her.

My daughter is ten months old and refuses to feed herself. Whenever we put food on the tray in front of her, she just picks it up and drops it over the edge of her high chair. We usually break down and feed her. What should we do?

I wouldn't do anything, except perhaps get a dog. She likely isn't ready or interested in feeding herself yet. This isn't a big problem since she has the rest of her life to feed herself. In the meantime, feed her as you usually would but try starting off one meal a day with a colorful, but small, selection of finger foods. If these morsels go to the dogs, don't react, since the novelty of your reaction and attention may be what's driving the behavior. Take a deep breath and move on to feeding her in the way that you normally would. One day she'll see the light and, believe it or not, actually get offended over the idea of you helping her.

My seven-month-old girl doesn't like to use a tippy cup. The baby books that I have say that she should be able to at this age. Should I be concerned?

Theoretically a baby should be able to drink from a tippy cup beginning around six or seven months. While this may be possible, not all babies are interested this early. In fact, some children will make it well into their second year without ever showing interest in anything but a bottle.

Try the following tips to help get things started:

- Continue to offer the tippy cup periodically without pressure or force. If she doesn't take it, put it away.
- Try offering diluted juice or water to create a novel drinking experience.
- Buy different varieties and colors—one may pique her interest and get things started.
- While holding your baby, try offering water or juice from a cup after you've drunk from it. Again, this may create a novel experience after which she may model her behavior.

DISCRIMINATING TASTES

My first child was an incredibly picky eater. What are the odds that I'll be facing the same thing with my second child?
Despite your worst fears, picky eating isn't considered a genetic problem. And as of the printing of this book, the picky gene has yet to be identified. While it may appear that your first child's penchant for pickiness couldn't possibly carry over to your second child, other factors besides genes may be involved. As with any disease or condition, the influence of the environment needs to be considered. Specifically, is there anything you may have done to promote picky feeding in your first child that may impact your second child in a similar way?

It may be oversimplifying things, however, to suggest that choosy toddlers are the way they are because of their parents. It simply isn't always the case. Some toddlers are tough to please despite all of the right moves on your part. This shouldn't stop you, however, from trying to assess how things went with your first child. Look through some of the questions in the remainder of the book and see how you could handle situations differently. Keep in mind, however, that no matter how much you read or how differently you do things, every child is different and her environment determines only part of who she ultimately becomes at the dinner table.

At what age does a child begin to show preferences for particular foods?

Children will begin to show preferences for particular foods as soon as they have the ability to turn their heads, close their mouths, or make foul faces, which is shortly after most babies start solids. What's important to remember about children is that their tastes and preferences can change as quickly as their diaper size. What's despised today may be part of next month's food jag. Avoid the temptation to declare your child as one who "hates" or "refuses" certain foods. Always leave the door open for a change of heart . . . or stomach.

At what age is it OK to begin seasoning a child's food?

Before you pass the salt and before I answer this one, ask yourself one question: Why are you interested in seasoning your baby's food?

- *Are you doing this to help a child eat?* This is a no-no. Don't use seasoning to try to get a child to eat a food that you think she might otherwise not be interested in. If you season food too early, children are likely to become dependent on particular flavors or tastes. Respect a child's disinterest in a food and don't apply your own seasoning preferences to get her to take something because you think she needs it. There is no one food a child can't live without.

- *Are you doing this because* you *don't like the way the food tastes?* This is also a no-no. What we give our children influences what they will prefer later on. If they are raised with unsalted food, it's likely that they'll never crave heavily salted food. While it may be inevitable, try not to

The Sweet Tooth: Born or Bred?

Are children born to love sugar, or is it our introduction of this intoxicating substance that makes tots crave it? The answer isn't well understood, although most experts would agree that it's probably a bit of both.

Our natural attraction to sweets can be found as early as the first few days of life. Studies done with newborns have demonstrated that they have the ability to discern sweetened from nonsweetened formula. Beyond the newborn period, there is evidence that the intensity of the response to a sweet taste varies from person to person. This has led experts to believe that some individuals do in fact harbor a "sweet tooth," or a true drive for sugar consumption.

This shouldn't serve as an excuse for our junk food compulsions, however. A child's preference for salt, sugar, and fat appears to be programmed early in life depending on what they're fed. And despite what we may know or have yet to learn about the biological drive for sugar, the environment children grow up in will always play a key role in how we eat as adults.

inflict your tastes and preferences on your child, especially when it involves potentially unhealthy condiments such as salt, butter, and extra sugar.

- *Are you doing this because it's normal and that's the way it's supposed to be eaten?* All seasoning is subjective and few foods need the seasoning that we provide. To deny a child from New Orleans the use of Tabasco sauce on his scrambled eggs is to deny an inevitable cultural norm and one that the child, or young adult, will ultimately catch on to. We can run but we can't hide. In the meantime, let your child become accustomed to the basic flavor before unleashing the world on his taste buds.

So when is it acceptable? The bottom line here is that seasoning, salting, buttering, and sweetening are reasonable once a child has established a varied palate on his own. So long as the child is old enough to understand that this isn't the only way a particular food tastes, it's reasonable to allow her to broaden her eating experience through seasoning. This may occur between four or five years. But remember, once you've had your eggs with Tabasco, it's hard to go back!

We tried to introduce baby food at five months to our daughter and she showed no interest in feeding from a spoon. Any cereal that we were able to get into her mouth immediately made its way down her bib. Thinking that she wasn't ready, we waited until seven months and nothing has changed. In fact, she appears even less interested now at eight months old. What's wrong?

Babies who are slow to pick up on spoon-feeding often are not given the chance to work on this important skill. More than likely, your baby had an exaggerated extrusor reflex, or the natural response to spit out all things solid. Those babies who seem insistent on spitting out their food usually need nothing more than a little time and gentle encouragement. In this case, the message that the parents heard was that the baby wasn't ready to feed. It is very unusual for a baby to not be ready for solids at five months.

The proper way to have handled this situation would have been to continue offering food (perhaps one to two teaspoons one to two times daily) despite the fact that she didn't seem to hold it in. This reflex usually goes away within a couple of weeks, and the feeding experience for both baby and parent improves dramatically. Unfortunately, this baby has now reached the ripe old age of eight months without any significant exposure to any form of baby food. She is well into the *texture zone*, or the period between six and ten months of age when children must learn to accept the texture and sensation that go along with solid food. The farther children get along in months, the more foreign the lumps and bumps of food will appear to them. The more foreign solid food appears to a baby, the less likely she is to happily smack and swallow. And this response only gets worse with time.

All is not lost in this case. The best way to handle it is to press on and feed the baby despite how she reacts. Offer two or three feedings a day of cereal or fruit and cereal—two or three teaspoons if that's all she'll tolerate. She's likely to dislike the whole process at first and object with crying and carrying on. Consider it training or a deconditioning exercise, which is really what it is. The key is gentle consistency; offer the feeds at each sitting but don't push the issue or create a stressful situation. If she begins to associate the high chair or spoon with anxiety or choking, you'll really be in trouble. Be patient. The rejection of solids in this case should begin to turn around in a few weeks.

Our twelve-month-old seems to enjoy throwing his tippy cup off of his high chair. Any advice?
The next time this happens, ignore it and give him one chance to correct himself by replacing the cup on the high chair. If he does it a second time, take the cup away and offer it after his feeding time is over. This is a case where your reaction to this frustrating problem drives the behavior. Give him the chance to use his tippy cup in the high chair but don't give him the pleasure of seeing you retrieve it.

EATING AND SLEEPING

What's the harm in letting a baby fall asleep with his bottle?
It seems parents will do just about anything to help their children settle down and fall asleep. And, unfortunately, the desperation involved in this process can lead some parents to start unhealthy, difficult-to-break habits. Bottle propping is one of them. Allowing a child to sleep with her bottle puts her at risk for the development of milk caries, or decay due to the prolonged bathing of milk against a baby's teeth. Some parents are under the misconception that this is OK if the bottle contains milk and not juice. This isn't true. Milk contains sugars that are just as destructive as those found in juice.

Offer a bottle only during waking hours when the teeth are protected by the irrigation that occurs with saliva and tongue movement. If it's a habit that you've already allowed your baby to get into, start by replacing the bottle contents with water to eliminate the destructive effects of sugar and then consider replacing the bottle with a pacifier. While this initially may not go over well, your baby will learn that it's easier to sleep than cry with or without a bottle.

My nine-month-old has begun crying in the middle of the night. We offer her a bottle and it seems to help. Does this mean she's not getting enough to eat during the day?

Most nine-month-olds are able to judge that they're getting enough to eat during the day such that they don't need to be fed at night. Infants at this age will experience what is referred to as "nighttime awakening." Whether awoken by a dream or distant barking dog, the idea of finding themselves alone and in the dark can be too much for most babies to handle. Some parents interpret these episodes of nighttime awakening as hunger, and the eager acceptance of a bottle reinforces that notion. After several nights of this, a baby will come to understand that her wailing leads not only to a midnight social break but also a warm bottle or cup.

Nighttime awakening is a normal event for children of this age. Be sure your baby has some familiar objects in her crib to help her understand that she's in a safe and familiar place. Let her cry. By all means, don't reinforce the behavior with food unless you're prepared to make nighttime visits a habit.

PEARLY WHITES

At what age should you begin brushing a baby's teeth?

While some disagree on the answer to this common question, the majority of child care and baby tooth experts recommend daily or every-other-day cleaning as soon as teeth make their appearance. When your baby's toothy grin is limited to one or two teeth, they can be wiped clean with a moist piece of gauze. Thereafter you should consider using a soft infant toothbrush. It not only does a more effective job, it will get your baby accustomed to a lifelong routine critical for the maintenance of a healthy smile.

How much should feeding be affected when a baby is cutting teeth?

Just before a tooth erupts, the overlying gum can be remarkably tender and children often will refuse everything but the softest food. Children in this situation often look and act as if hungry but pull away and cry when offered their favorite table food. If you see this behavior along with the characteristic finger chewing, drooling, and swollen gums, it's safe to assume that the behavior is a consequence of teething. You may consider regressing to soft or pureed foods such as applesauce, gelatin, or pudding—chilled, if possible. These will satisfy your baby's hunger and provoke her gums the least. This sensitive feeding behavior should last no more than four or five days (assuming there's only one tooth coming in at a time!) but may carry on for a couple of weeks if the child has a good memory.

My daughter is nine months old and doesn't have any teeth. Is this a problem and is there anything we can do to promote her teeth coming in?

Assuming that your child is an otherwise happy, healthy nine-month-old, you'll need to be patient. The timing of tooth eruption is tied most closely to genetic factors, such as

---

Preemie Teeth—Fashionably Late

They may have arrived early but their teeth are usually late. On average, infants born premature begin to show their primary teeth three months later than babies born at term. Remember that tooth development begins as early as two months after conception and continues right up until they make their appearance, but the stress of preemie life affects how those teeth develop. It has been theorized that delayed tooth eruption in former prematures depends on the degree of prematurity, length of time on a breathing machine, and amount of time baby goes without all of her nutrition by gut.

And former prematures aren't out of the woods when their teeth appear. It has been shown that the formation of their tooth enamel (the protective outer coating of the tooth) is often poor. This makes them easy targets for tooth decay.

when Mom or Dad sprouted teeth. Unfortunately, there's no fertilizer available for teeth.

While it's quite unusual for term infants to go beyond a year without teeth, it can indicate an underlying problem. It's up to your pediatrician to look at your baby's overall growth, development, and nutritional status to determine whether further evaluation or just more patience is indicated.

Does teething cause diarrhea?

While many parents have reported loose stools or diarrhea during the throes of teething, it has never been proven with any controlled studies. While it's hard to connect tooth eruption with stool consistency, it makes more sense to look at the other things that are going on during periods of teething. It has been theorized that the excessive salivation of teething may play a role in this phenomenon. Saliva is abundant in enzymes that play a small but important role in digestion. And anyone who's ever cared for a teething child understands that his diet can make brief and dramatic changes that may impact on number two.

When should an infant begin to receive fluoride supplementation?

It is recommended that breast-fed infants and those fed formula without supplemented water (ready-to-feed and concentrate prepared with bottle water or nonsupplemented tap water) receive 0.25 mg of fluoride per day after six months of age.

How do I find out the fluoride content of our municipal water supply?

This information should be available from your local town hall. Usually parents can call a hot line or the office of water quality to learn the level of fluoride in their local water. Understand that levels may vary from one part of town to the other so be prepared to give your crossroads or zip code.

Checking for Fluoride in Your Water

Tap water may not provide what your child needs for optimal dental health. According to the Centers for Disease Control and Prevention (CDC) Fluoridation Census, less than two-thirds of the U.S. population has a fluoridated water supply. To see if your child is receiving the fluoride she needs, check out the following table and talk to your pediatrician or dentist about supplementation.

If your muninicipal water supply provides . . .

	LESS THAN 0.3 PPM F	0.3–0.6 PPM F	MORE THAN 0.6 PPM F
You'll need to provide your child with . . .			
Birth–6 months	0	0	0
6 months–3 years	0.25 mg	0	0
3–6 years	0.50 mg	0.25 mg	0
6–16 years	1 mg	0.50 mg	0

I've heard that ready-to-feed infant formula contains fluoride. Is this true?

While some infant formula manufacturers supplemented their products with fluoride in the past, most products currently contain no fluoride. Be sure to check with your pediatrician or the manufacturer of your child's formula.

When should a child have her first visit to the dentist?

It depends on whom you ask. Pediatric dentists suggest that a child have her first visit to the dentist by one year old. The dentists are most concerned about preventive maintenance and early initiation of healthy dental habits. Most pediatricians feel that a child can wait until her third birthday before first visiting the dentist.

Too Much of a Good Thing?

When it comes to toothpaste and babies, more is definitely *not* better. Any toothpaste used in excess of what's absolutely necessary may get swallowed. And if there are other sources of fluoride in a child's diet, such as through a vitamin or municipal water supply, this excessive intake can lead to stained teeth due to a condition known as fluorosis. When brushing a baby's teeth, use a very tiny amount, about the size of half of a pencil eraser.

SPOONS, CUPS, AND CHAIRS—
THE FEEDING ENVIRONMENT

At what age should a baby begin using a high chair?

A baby can begin to use a high chair as soon as she is able to sit on her own with support. If you've chosen to feed your baby before she can be comfortably perched in a high chair, you can feed her seated in your lap. If you have a high chair that reclines, you can use this. But remember that one of the signs of solid readiness is (among other things) a baby's ability to support her own head. Anything more than a slight recline is unnatural and makes it difficult to spit out food that she may not be able to handle at any given moment.

A Few Words About High Chairs

To parents, a baby's move to the high chair represents an exciting new phase in their feeding development. To babies, the high chair represents "time to eat." This association of their high, cockpitlike position with the need to do business is an important one. The anticipation of eating triggered by the high chair sets a variety of necessary intestinal processes in motion, including salivation and production of stomach acid. And while eating should be fun, children must learn early on that this is where they come to eat. Consider the following points when choosing a high chair:

- While it may be hard to conceive of when you're purchasing your first high chair, remember that your baby ultimately will make the transition to eating with you at the table. When that time comes it's nice to have a chair with a removable tray that can be adjusted to the height of your kitchen table. This will make the transition easier and may allow you to skip a booster seat altogether.
- While there are chairs available with attached toys and distractions, remember that high chairs should be reserved for eating and should not be a place for fun and entertainment.
- Make sure that you can control the tray with one hand. In most cases your other hand will be occupied with a spaghetti-covered baby or wet wipe.
- Most features are constant from chair to chair. Some are required by law and the rest are personal preference.

Why are feeder bottles considered taboo?

What's more frightening than the fact that these contraptions can be found in stores is that there's a market driving their demand. For those not familiar with them, feeder bottles are devices that allow solid food, in combination with milk, to be sluiced through a nipplelike appliance into a baby's mouth. Feeder bottles should be considered evil. They promote overfeeding and prevent developmentally appropriate feeding habits. Until these things go the way of evaporated milk and leeches, stick with a bowl and spoon.

Chapter 6

Toddlerhood and Beyond

The twelve-to-thirty-six-month age group represents one of the most challenging times for feeding a child. It's now that children begin to achieve independence and their tastes become more particular. Part of the problem with feeding the toddler is that he is advanced enough to control what goes into his mouth, but he's not advanced enough to be reasoned with or know what's in his best interest. Even outside the high chair, it's important to understand the fine line between enforcing appropriate behavior and allowing a toddler to express developmentally appropriate behavior. Understanding your role isn't easy. The firm limits you set as a parent are just as critical as the free license you give your child to experiment with and refuse the food that's provided. You're in a tough position, and self-doubt is normal for parents.

To understand the problems you may encounter while feeding toddlers, it's important to understand their issues and what makes them tick. Only then can you come to accept what they'll do (or not do) at the high chair. A thorough understanding of what's normal will help you accept your child's behavior and feel less responsible for her seemingly irrational, quirky actions. I once had a mother point out to me that feeding toddlers takes a lot of negotiating—they've got their own strong ideas about everything, they're impulsive, there are no rules, and it's tough to make them change. The only way to get through this trying period without disaster is to work with them and, to some extent, play by their rules.

Perhaps the most important underlying principle in successful toddler feeding is the *division of responsibility*. This simple concept, first popularized by feeding therapist Ellyn Satter, stipulates that you as a parent are responsible for providing food to your child and she in turn is responsible for eating it. That's it, no exceptions. What's so important about this simple idea is that it frees parents from the common misunderstanding that they're responsible for what their kids do. It's this misunderstanding that leads parents to bribe, coax, and even try to force-feed their toddler—all nasty little habits that lead to maladaptive feeding relationships. When children are left on their own to do what they do best, they'll usually surprise us. It's an amazingly simple idea and one that, if more widely accepted, would change the way we see toddlers and how they feed.

THE QUESTION OF MILK

When can children begin to take regular cow's milk?

Cow's milk should be withheld until a child is twelve months old. The premature introduction of cow's milk to infants can lead to irritation of the bowel lining and mild but chronic blood loss. After one year your child's digestive system will be better able to tolerate the level of protein and minerals found in cow's milk. Keep in mind that there's no reason to offer your child cow's milk any sooner. If breast-feeding, you should be striving to reach at least this age before weaning. For non–breast-fed infants, formulas are designed to provide most of what a baby needs through the first year.

How much milk should my toddler be drinking?

Toddlers and preschoolers should take in approximately sixteen to twenty-four ounces of milk a day. For a solid eater, her needs may be met with fewer than sixteen ounces. For the choosy eater, milk may represent over half of her calorie intake, and an amount closer to the upper end of that range may be best.

Is it OK to give my toddler low-fat milk?

It's recommended that toddlers between the ages of twelve and twenty-four months receive whole milk. This is because for most children this age, milk continues to represent a significant source of protein and calories. Skim milk should be avoided since its watery consistency tends to promote increased consumption by thirsty toddlers. This can lead to excess intake of protein, which can be harmful to the kidneys.

My son is a year old and he was diagnosed with milk allergy at six weeks. Since then he has been on Alimentum (casein hydrolysate formula). Can he be put on regular cow's milk at this age, or does he first need to be put on a standard infant formula?

Parents are always anxious when it comes to advancing their previously allergic baby on to regular milk. The fact is that the majority of babies with a history of milk protein hypersensitivity are fine by their first birthday. They should be able to advance on to whole milk as any normal toddler. If your baby experienced unusually severe symptoms of milk allergy as an infant with excessive bleeding, diarrhea, eczematous rash, and breathing symptoms, you should talk to your pediatrician or gastroenterologist before taking this step. Sometimes in this setting a formal milk challenge is recommended. In a milk challenge a child is slowly given small amounts of milk under close monitoring in a hospital setting. This allows for support in the event that a severe reaction takes place.

My toddler refuses to drink milk. What should I do and can you recommend alternative sources of calcium?

Despite what's drilled into our head by the advertising executives on Madison Avenue, children can live without milk. The reason we like milk is that it provides a convenient source of calories, protein, and calcium all in one form that can be taken from a bottle or tippy cup. It's especially important for those children who are picky eaters since it may represent the majority of their nutritional intake. For those children, milk is very helpful for proper growth and development.

If your child refuses to drink milk, the first issue to address is why. It may be that she's become used to breast milk or formula from her bottle. Sometimes this presents a great opportunity to start her on a tippy cup. It could be that she's become accustomed to other, more appealing, options, such as juice. In this case you may want to make her milk cup the only option perhaps in the morning and with dinner.

Sources of Calcium
Calcium-processed tofu
Blackstrap molasses
Calcium-fortified orange juice
Dried figs
Cottage cheese
Fortified cereals
Yogurt
Leafy green vegetables (mustard greens and broccoli)

When there's nothing else to drink, a cup of milk may start to look good after a half hour or so. Set the cup on a step stool or other accessible place and you'll be surprised. Once the child learns that her options are limited, the juice-seeking will likely disappear within a few days.

Despite your best efforts, there are children who will not drink milk. If your child eats like a horse, she can live without milk, but you'll need to find alternate calcium sources to make up for lost milk. These include yogurt, cheddar cheese, calcium-fortified orange juice, cottage cheese, and fortified cereals. And don't look to a multivitamin to cover what she's not getting from her milk. Most children's multivitamins don't contain calcium. If she eats like a bird, you'll need to supplement calories *and* calcium. This child is at risk nutritionally and should be followed by a pediatric dietician to ensure that her needs are met.

Is it OK to give my fourteen-month-old chocolate milk if she refuses regular milk?

While it's never a good idea to make a habit of using sweetening, seasoning, or flavoring as a means of getting a child to eat, flavored milk may save the picky eater who isn't keen on the plain stuff. Milk represents such a valuable source of protein and calories that the nutritional benefit outweighs any transient habits that may develop with flavoring. Try to avoid flavored milks in the dairy case that are made with low-fat milk. Use chocolate or strawberry *whole* milk or prepare your own by adding flavored powder. Milk-based smoothies concocted in the blender with frozen strawberries and yogurt may go over well when faced with a stalemate.

Does my baby need a toddler formula?

Toddler, or transitional, formulas are nutritional supplements intended to take over where infant formulas leave off. When compared with whole milk, transitional formulas contain more appropriate levels of protein and higher amounts of essential vitamins and minerals, such as vitamins E and C, niacin, and iron. Although they may seem ideal, they may not be necessary for a child with a balanced diet. Beginning in the second year of life, a toddler's diet expands to contain foods high in all of the nutrients necessary for growth. You may want to check with your pediatrician about using a toddler formula—especially if your toddler is an unusually picky eater or doesn't like milk.

My two-year-old is obsessed with milk. He drinks forty ounces a day. Despite our best attempts to offer alternatives, he insists on milk. Is this a problem?

Unless a child is constipated or drinking milk exclusive of other foods, a fixation with milk shouldn't be a problem. Some children are provided with cups or bottles of milk throughout the day and allowed to graze at will. This is likely to interfere with a child's appetite and normal drive to eat. At this age drinks of any sort, including milk, should be provided around a basic schedule of three meals a day and two snacks. The concern here is that milk may be taking the place of other foods that make up a balanced toddler diet. Assuming the normal up-and-down variations of a toddler diet, he shouldn't need more than twenty ounces of milk a day to meet his minimal needs for protein and calcium.

In this case, offer milk with meals, perhaps eight ounces three times a day. Be sure to offer the milk once he's gotten a good start on the meal. Water or diluted juice will add variety at snack time (two to three times a day) and prevent him from filling up. If he refuses to drink either of these, don't provide alternatives. In time he'll decide to drink or go thirsty. A child has yet to become dehydrated from refusing water.

How can I tell if my child is lactose intolerant?

Lots of parents report lactose intolerance and problems with dairy products in their children, but true lactose intolerance (or loss of the enzyme that digests milk sugar) is actually quite uncommon before the school-age years. Symptoms of lactose intolerance include crampy abdominal pain, bloating, gas, and diarrhea. These may occur hours after drinking milk when the ingested lactose, unabsorbed in the small intestine, makes its way into the colon, where it is eaten by the bacteria that live there. The result is diarrhea and gas.

While taking your child off of dairy products may seem like a good way to test your lactose intolerance hypothesis, this method is flawed. Lactose is hidden in a wide variety of prepared foods. Some pancake mixes, for example, contain significant amounts of lactose and can foil a test for lactose intolerance. If you're truly concerned about the possibility of lactose intolerance in your toddler, talk to your doctor or see a pediatric gastroenterologist.

Can lactose intolerance be tested for in children?

There is a test for lactose intolerance more scientific than withholding milk. It's called a *lactose breath test*. This test is usually performed by a pediatric gastroenterologist, a specialist in children's digestive disorders. In this test, the child is given a drink containing a certain amount of lactose. For the two to three hours following the drink, periodic samples of the child's breath are taken and measured for changes in hydrogen level. Marked changes in breath hydrogen after an hour or so into the test indicate that the undigested lactose has made its way into the colon and is under fermentation by the bacteria that live there.

How is organic milk different from regular milk?

The term "organic milk" suggests that the farm involved with raising the cows used no man-made fertilizer, hormones, pesticides, or antibiotics in either the livestock or their feed. While more costly, the nutritional value of the milk itself shouldn't differ.

Our family has recently begun drinking soy milk in place of regular milk as part of a new heart-healthy diet. Is this safe for our four-year-old?

Yes, soy milk is a safe milk alternative for children. And while it may not be absolutely necessary to a child's well-being, milk of any variety happens to be a convenient way to deliver calories and protein to kids. There are differences, however, between the two types of milk. Compared with cow's milk, soy contains about 30 percent less protein and falls short on vitamin A, vitamin B12, folate, zinc, and calcium. Many brands of soy milk fortify with vitamin B12 and calcium, making this a moot point. The differences become even less important if your child is taking a reasonable variety of other foods.

Aside from being a source of protein and vitamins, soy milk has the advantage of containing less saturated fat than cow's milk and no cholesterol. It is rich in phytoestrogens, which may play a role in preventing certain types of cancer. Soy milk contains no lactose, although this should have little impact on most children since true lactose intolerance is very uncommon until well into the school-age years.

FOOD FIGHTS

My two-year-old is very picky about what he likes to eat. Even though the pediatrician tells me he is growing, I'm absolutely certain that no one could live on the amount my son takes in. Should I find another pediatrician?

If you find another pediatrician, he or she will look at the same growth curve and, it is hoped, come to the same conclusion that your two-year-old is doing just fine. Growth curves don't lie, and the basic deviations in growth that children experience on their way to adulthood aren't open to a whole lot of interpretation. Your experience is very common, however—parents often are shocked to find that their child has gained weight on a diet that seems limited to Fruit Roll-Ups and bologna. Toddlers achieve appropriate intake of calories and various nutrients over time. When you look at your toddler's diet, it's important to look at his intake over a matter of *days to weeks* rather than from *meal to meal*. A formal calculation of food eaten over the long run would show that most toddlers, especially those with normal growth, eat what they need when they need it.

One last thought on changing pediatricians: Perhaps you don't feel confident in the way your concerns are being addressed. It may be time to find a new pediatrician on that basis alone.

My toddler seems to have a fixation with macaroni and cheese. Is there any way to break her of this?

This may represent a preference that you happen to be feeding in to (no pun intended) or a true food jag where your child is transiently obsessed with the color, consistency, or appearance of mac and cheese to the exclusion of all other foods. Food jags are the trademark of the toddler feeding experience, and unfortunately there's little you can do once they're under way.

While it may be hard and even pointless to try to break your child of her food jag, it doesn't mean that you can't head one off before it occurs. Consider these pointers:

- Be sure to offer a small variety of two or three different foods at each meal to allow your child some degree of control and choice in her feeding decisions.

- If your child thumbs her nose at the options presented, offer no alternative. Remember Ellyn Satter's division of responsibility: You're responsible only for what's presented; your child is responsible for eating it.

- Don't offer alternatives for fear that she'll go hungry or become malnourished. This will almost always lead to a pattern of choosy behavior and whining.

- Consider exploiting her fixation by adding small amounts of chopped cooked broccoli, diced zucchini, carrots, or chicken to her macaroni and cheese.

What Should My Child Be Eating?

While it's difficult to come up with anything typical for a toddler, these menu selections are an example of what a one- to two-year-old might eat on any given day. Three meals a day with a mid-morning and late-afternoon snack is typical. Meals should be taken with six to eight ounces of milk.

Breakfast
½ cup of oatmeal or iron-fortified cereal
½ banana
OR
Frozen waffle with yogurt on top
2 cleaned, diced strawberries

Snack
Thick pear or apple slices spread with soft, flavored cream cheese
OR
1 graham cracker with peanut butter spread thin

Lunch
½ egg salad sandwich
½ cup of applesauce
OR
½ grilled cheese sandwich cut in strips
Thin wedge of cantaloupe

Dinner
⅓ cup of cooked elbow macaroni with 1 tablespoon of spaghetti sauce and ¼ cup of shredded zucchini
OR
½ cup cooked brown rice with ⅓ cup black beans and finely shredded chicken breast

My two-and-a-half-year-old is a picky eater, and I struggle to get her to take even a few bites. If she refuses food at the dinner table, should I prepare something else for her?

This is one of the greatest dilemmas faced by parents. *If she doesn't eat she'll starve but if I give in maybe I'm contributing to some sort of bad habit.* The fact is that falling short on a meal or two will not cause starvation. However, meeting her demand for some alternative that she finds more appealing at that moment sets a dangerous precedent. Once children realize that they have a short-order cook in the house, they won't hesitate to have it their way. Stick to the routine of providing two or three appealing foods at a sitting and let her decide how hungry she really is.

The exception to this is when a child is faced with pain from teething or an ear infection. In this case certain solid foods will be extremely painful, and you may notice your child begin to bite her food only to spit it out. In this case it's reasonable to provide a soft, soothing alternative, such as yogurt or diced fruit.

My thirty-month-old is an incredibly picky eater who has been small (but growing) all of her life. She refuses most foods except cheese puffs, breakfast bars, cookies, and a few other less-than-healthy choices. If we don't offer her these she won't eat at all and we think that, given her size, it's better for her to get calories from junk food than not at all. Is this sound reasoning?

This is the old *give-me-cookies-or-watch-me-starve* routine. It's been around as long as parenthood itself, and it's perhaps the most common dilemma among parents of thin, picky children. Is junk food better than no food? As a general rule, no. The weakness in the argument lies in the belief that "no food" is dangerous, especially for a child barely hanging on to the growth curve. Most parents get caught in this quagmire of twisted logic when they're faced with a child they perceive as sick. But lean, picky children should be seen only as lean, picky children and not sick children with free license to eat what they wish on their terms. In

---

Satter's Division of Responsibility

If you don't take anything else away from this book, please take away an understanding of Satter's division of responsibility. This landmark concept in childhood feeding first popularized by feeding therapist Ellyn Satter states very simply that *parents* are responsible for what's provided and *children* are responsible for what's eaten. In other words, your responsibility as a parent should be to provide a tempting variety of appealing, nutritious foods for your toddler. How much winds up being eaten is up to your child.

Most parents have a very difficult time with this. After all, toddlers are supposed to be finicky, picky eaters, and part of parenthood is the conning and negotiating that goes on at the high chair. Making food into a zooming airplane and successfully feeding a moving target is part of what it takes to keep our kids healthy and nourished, right? Wrong. Children know what they want and when. And as frustrating as it may seem, we should respect their cues for hunger and foster healthy habits early on.

Try to see the division of responsibility as means of liberating you from the stress and concern that may be keeping you a captive to the high chair at mealtime. This detachment from what your independent toddler does with her food is key to successful feeding while overinvolvement is key to the development of feeding struggles.

---

most situations like the one you have described, the child is playing the parent like a dime store ukulele. Most parents wind up far down the primrose path lured on by the threat of failure to thrive, brain damage, or whatever horrible outcome they imagine from a skipped meal or two.

This is a situation that can be remedied only by reassurance with the facts. And the fact is that the child who's small and growing is typically nothing to be concerned about. The child who's small but not growing, on the other hand, is always something to be concerned about. A pediatrician or pediatric gastroenterologist should closely monitor the situation, usually with the input of an experienced pediatric dietician. A dietician will sometimes encourage certain high-calorie foods to improve energy intake, but never junk food. If you're not sure that there's even a problem with your child's growth, get the facts so that you can comfortably enforce the division of responsibility and finally bring order back to the high chair.

At what age should a child be expected to behave at the table?
One of the great misconceptions about children is that they
are naturally unruly, mischievous, and difficult to control. This
apathetic attitude adopted by some parents creates a self-ful-
filling prophecy that allows for inappropriate behavior.

Reactive Feeding Anxiety: The Seed of the Feeding Struggle

THE PROBLEM

How do we get into problems feeding our children and how does it all start?
Are children born to be picky eaters, or is it something we do to set these behaviors in motion? While it's hard to say for sure, the problems that we face
feeding our children are probably a consequence of both. But how we look at
feeding as parents may be very different from how our kids see it. Children, by
nature, have no fear of eating. While skeptical and quirky at times, most are naturally curious and adventurous at the high chair. Parents, on the other hand, are
notorious for having fears and issues about how their kids eat. What parents often overlook is the powerful role this fear can play in a child's relationship with
her food.

   This leads us to a concept that I refer to as *reactive feeding anxiety*. This
idea simply states that behavioral feeding difficulties are often the consequence
of the way a parent reacts to a child's behavior. What may be a developmentally
appropriate way for a child to respond to her food may be misinterpreted as
problematic. This reaction by the parent initiates stress in the feeding relationship that ultimately affects how the child is fed. So while we can't control the
way our children are, we can control the way we respond to what they do. In this
respect, feeding problems may be more a result of what we do as parents.

THE FAULTY THOUGHT PROCESS

To make the whole concept easier to visualize, consider the following thoughts
and reactions that illustrate reactive feeding anxiety:

- Parent sees child refusing food.
- Parent becomes anxious over the fear that the food is critical to the child's
  health.
- Reacting to what's perceived as a critical situation, parent tries to feed child
  by any means possible, including coercion, threats, and subtle force-feeding.
- The child (1) remembers the attention that this game draws or (2) becomes
  anxious over being forced to eat when his body isn't ready to be fed. In either
  case, the child is likely to perpetuate this behavior at the next meal, which in
  (continued)

turn generates more anxiety and draws a more intense reaction from parent. And so it goes.

For those of you who have already read this book, this scenario is flawed at every step.

- *Children frequently refuse to eat from time to time.*
- *No one meal is ever critical enough to warrant divisive feeding tactics.*
- *Coercion at the high chair nearly always leads to problems.*

UNDERSTANDING YOUR WAY OUT

The beauty of this problem is that it's fairly easy to fix since it assumes you're the only party in the feeding relationship with a problem. While your child's disrupted feeding pattern may require some time to get healthy again, some simple adjustments in your feeding perspective is all that's needed to get back on the straight and narrow. To prevent this you have to:

- *Understand what's developmentally and behaviorally appropriate for your child's age.* In other words, what's normal. What are the quirks that toddlers or infants bring to the high chair that are normal and healthy? This can come from reading books like this, talking to your pediatrician, and finding a good feeding role model.
- *Understand the basics of toddler nutrition.* In other words, understand what you can get away with and what's dangerous. In most cases, parents overstate the importance of a particular meal or food to the point that a struggle ensues. In the big picture this sort of struggle leads to greater problems than missing a single meal.
- *Understand your child and yourself.* With a basic understanding of what's normal for other kids, you'll need to learn what works for your child. What are her quirks and idiosyncrasies, and how can you work around these in a healthy way? Almost more important than knowing your child is knowing yourself and your own fears.

The problems that children have feeding are often the consequence of what we do as parents. While no one intentionally does things to keep their child from eating well, it's important to understand our role in the process and what we can do about it. It's our response to what children do and don't do that sets the mood of our feeding relationship.

How you enforce behavior at the table probably will have a lot to do with how you enforced behavior in the high chair. And how you enforce behavior in the high chair is closely related to how you handle things throughout the day. How you handle the broader issue of limit setting with your child is beyond the scope of this book, but consider the following guidelines to create better behavior at the table:

- She should understand from early on that certain behaviors, such as screeching, are not tolerated at the table.
- Mealtime is not playtime, and toys should not be allowed at the high chair.
- Meals should be started and finished at the table.
- Meals have a definite beginning and an end.
- Dinnertime is not TV time. Avoid the mesmerizing dependency of the television to facilitate eating.
- The meal is not centered around her and should (at least once a day) be a family time. Ultimately she should understand that what's prepared for the family is what the family eats despite her wishes for chicken fingers or macaroni and cheese.

Children should be expected to behave at the table just as soon as they're able to sit up. Remember that the limits of your child's behavior are determined early on, and table manners should be no exception.

Our son is fourteen months old and he takes table food only with encouragement. He recently cut two molars, and during that time refused to take anything but baby food. We went along with it over concerns that he would go hungry, but now he refuses table food knowing we'll probably give in. What should we do?
While teething can cause a temporary aversion to solids, it shouldn't last for more than a week or two. In this case you'll need to draw the line once it's clear that the teething issue is passed. Try gradually mixing small amounts of solid food with his favorite baby food. Bits of pasta or steamed veggies add texture and variety and may raise his curiosity for other advanced foods. Slowly increase the amount of table food so that it replaces the baby food over a couple of weeks.

My eighteen-month-old seems to have a fixation with crunchy foods. We have no problem getting him to eat oat cereal, cheese crackers, or the crust off chicken nuggets. He refuses cheese and other soft items. What's going on?

Toddlers often demonstrate preferences for certain types and textures of food. Most often it's purely toddler prerogative and nothing more than a quirk of the age. In other cases it can represent what's referred to as an oral aversion, or a hypersensitive panic response to a particular texture. If the exposure to cheesy or slippery textures is accompanied by gagging or other significant signs of protest, it may represent a true oral aversion. You may want to talk to your doctor about a referral to a good pediatric occupational therapist for a period of therapy to try to get him over this. Otherwise you're probably facing nothing more than a frustrating by-product of toddlerhood that will go away with time and the proper variety of foods.

Safe at the Plate: Foods for Toddlers to Avoid

Always watch children during meals and snacks. Young children, ages two to three, are at an especially high risk of choking and remain at risk until they can chew and swallow better around age four. This is a partial list of potentially dangerous foods:

Hot dog (quartered lengthwise, then diced)
Whole grapes
Raisins
Nuts
Popcorn
Marshmallows
Hard candy
Chips and pretzels
Raw carrots
Thickly spread peanut butter

Our daughter is nineteen months old and will take table food only if it's dabbed with applesauce. Is this a habit we should try to break or is it just a phase?

I'm not sure what constitutes a "phase," but this sure sounds like one. While it's typically not a good idea to sweeten or season food as a condition for eating, this certainly sounds like a simple maneuver to keep the peace and it's unlikely to become a lifelong habit. It's also likely your daughter is as enraptured with the appearance of applesauce or the act of you

---

Creating Opportunities

Rather than looking at meals and snacks as defined times during which your toddler must eat, see them instead as opportunities for sampling, tasting, and experimenting with new flavors and textures. While your baby may not take advantage of every meal that comes her way, remember it's opportunity that creates possibility. Relaxing and letting your child decide which opportunities she'll take advantage of and which she'll turn away can have dramatic results.

---

dabbing the food as she is with its sweet taste. Just like dealing with the typical toddler food jag, be sure to offer variety. Consider using different sauces for dipping, such as yogurt, and try allowing her to get involved with the process.

Our eighteen-month-old refuses all vegetables. Any advice?

While vegetables are part of a balanced diet, keep in mind that toddlers very often go through periods of extreme imbalance in their feeding. On any given day, any given toddler may seem to have a dangerously restricted diet. This may seem scary, but it's normal. Don't let this evolve into a pressure situation at the high chair. Give your child options and never attempt to put food where it isn't wanted.

If it's imperative that you see your child eating zucchini or squash, you may need to get creative with your presentation. Like some adults, toddlers are remarkably particular about the way things look on their plate. Simply altering your recipes to disguise the vegetable in question is often enough to address your vegetable anxiety and provide a little more balance in your toddler's diet. For great toddler recipes, see Bridget Swinney's book *Healthy Foods for Healthy Kids* (New York: Meadowbrook Press, 1999). It's packed with creative recipes that address this very issue.

Consider the following suggestions on this timeless dilemma:

- *Don't sweat it.* Don't tell anyone you read it here, but the importance of vegetables to toddlers is probably overrated. As long as you're providing a balance of other foods such as fruits, you're OK.

- *Get off her back . . . or high chair.* If you don't take anything else away from this book, please take away the fact that pressure doesn't work. Struggles over any sort of food, especially peas and brussels sprouts, won't get you anywhere. If you get caught holding the spoon, ask yourself one question: "Twenty years from now, will this serving of peas have any impact on her life?"

- *Be patient.* New foods take time. Believe it or not, some researchers have counted the number of times children were offered unfamiliar food before trying them. On average, the children were exposed to a food eight times before they ate it.

- *Be manipulative and underhanded.* If you have to get those veggies in, consider covert measures. While I normally don't condone sneaky and divisive feeding tactics, it may be reasonable in this situation. Try mincing in broccoli with her mac and cheese or zucchini with her favorite lasagna. What she doesn't know might help her.

- *Change the format.* Offer variety in terms of color, size, shape, and texture. Finger-fed carrot sticks with a yogurt dip may be better received than overcooked diced carrots fed with a spoon. The novelty angle often works wonders when it comes to a feeding stalemate.

- *Be a role model.* Set an example for your children. Do you eat vegetables? Most young children try to model themselves after their parents. Those carrots on your child's plate will likely go uneaten if they are left on your plate. Kids notice what their mommies and daddies are doing.

Our seventeen-month-old loves meat, but he is slow to swallow it. He will chew for up to ten minutes, and sometimes we have to wash it down with mushy foods or milk. Is this normal?
This is entirely normal. Meat and chicken represent relatively tough foods that require more intense chewing than the cut fruit and pasta that make up most of the toddler diet. Meat is also swallowed in a fairly solid form, which is also a new concept for your son and one that will take some getting

used to. Keep in mind that his molars may not be in until eighteen to twenty-four months, and these are key meat-chewing teeth. Even then, meat and poultry should be well cooked, moist, and finely chopped. While frustrating, all you can do is let him work it out and help things along as you have done.

As a variation on this theme, some children will chew and never swallow, only to spit the meat out after a while. If this occurs, don't make a big deal out of it. It just means that they're probably not quite ready. Be sure the meat is prepared properly and continue to offer it from time to time so that they get used to the texture of meat and the concept of chewing it.

My child refuses to eat meat. Is he getting enough protein?

Inadequate protein intake is rare in children who are not strict vegetarians. If your child is growing normally, he is very likely eating the protein he needs. Foods other than meat that are high in protein include milk, yogurt, cheese, peanut butter, and eggs. While this feeding quirk is very common for children under the age of three or four, keep offering small amounts of well-cooked, well-cut-up meat on a consistent basis and it should pass.

My two-year-old often refuses to eat her macaroni and cheese if it's touching any one of the vegetables on her plate. Her peanut butter and jelly sandwiches also have to be cut into triangles before she'll consider eating them. Is this normal? We want her to eat but we don't want to create a spoiled child.

As crazy and irrational as it may seem, what you've described is normal feeding behavior for a two-year-old. In fact, it represents the developmentally healthy interest that toddlers have in controlling their environment. As frustrating as it may seem, keep in mind that this isn't a consequence of anything you've done and it's temporary.

While it's OK to conform to what seems to be a rigid way of having things, keep in mind that she may not know what she really wants and her quirks can change from day to day. Try to accommodate her within reason and then understand that whether she eats or not is out of your hands. Tantrums over their own frustration are common among toddlers, and understanding where to draw the line as a parent can be difficult. Remember Satter's division of responsibility: You're responsible for what's provided (and sometimes its shape), and your child is responsible for what's eaten.

It's All in the Delivery

Toddlers are characteristically fickle about the appearance, shape, and size of what's put in front of them. And much of what a toddler does with her food has to do with the way it's presented to them. Consider the following tips when presenting food to your toddler:

- Introduce new foods with another familiar food alongside it.
- Don't offer too much food or too many options. Toddlers easily become overwhelmed when faced with too much food or too many to choose from. Variety is key but limit options to two to three at any given meal.
- Prepare your child's food to meet her wishes. Trimming the edges from a sandwich or leaving a banana whole to keep the peace and encourage eating is perfectly appropriate. It shouldn't be considered giving in or spoiling your child. Be forewarned, though, that today's fickle fetish is the source of tomorrow's meltdown—a toddler's preferences can change rather quickly.

Our four-year-old is very picky and when eating out, he insists on chicken strips only. If he doesn't get chicken strips, he doesn't eat and only picks at other options given to him. This has limited our choice of restaurants. How should we deal with this? Your child's refusal to eat anything besides chicken fingers is his problem, not yours. And it sounds like you've been propagating this behavior by only choosing chicken-finger–dispensing restaurants. If he chooses to refuse one of the several appealing choices available on most children's menus, let him go hungry and tolerate no whining. As hard as it may seem in the short term, your subsequent dining encounters (sans chicken fingers) should go smoothly.

If our daughter doesn't have a good meal or refuses to eat what we give her, we typically withhold dessert. Does this sort of punishment work?

I wouldn't refer to this as punishment but rather a consistent approach to developing balanced eating habits early on. Toddlers don't have a sense of what constitutes a balanced diet, and they need our guidance to help determine what sorts of things are best eaten and when. If a child knows every meal ends with cookies, she may very well choose to skip the first course or two knowing what's coming. This sort of choosy behavior doesn't fly.

> ### "Winning the Food Wars"
>
> One of the latest feeding books urges parents in its subheading to "win the food wars." Any book that suggests that feeding is a battle shouldn't be trusted. While firm limits are fine, it's important to understand that there are undeniable quirks that represent your child's evolving independence and search for control. Fighting these normal developmental issues is futile. You won't win and any view of the high chair as a battleground will undoubtedly be met with casualties.

Knowing when a child has put her best foot forward is something that only you can decide. As a general rule, provide two or three options on a toddler's plate with the understanding that she'll dig into one or two of them. These should include foods that the rest of the family is eating. If she makes the effort to eat one or two of the nutritious foods that everyone else at the table has come to accept, then dessert is a reasonable option.

Some feeding experts see this as rewarding a child for eating something that her body may not want. I say that if her body doesn't want at least one of the three nutritious options that you provide, it certainly can't want dessert either. Don't bend on this one.

Our four-year-old has been followed by a pediatric gastroenterologist for poor eating and marginal growth. We've scraped by with supplements and high-calorie foods that have kept her growing, but she's still smaller than other kids her age. She recently began preschool and her eating has improved

dramatically. While we're excited about her new appetite, does this mean we've been doing something wrong at home?

While struggles with choosy eaters are almost epidemic in households with toddlers, most children take in adequate calories over the course of days to weeks to ensure normal growth. There are, however, other children who are consistently choosy and fail to take in the energy and nutrients to grow at a normal rate. In other words, these are children who won't eat and won't grow. The children who fall under this category of poor growth fail to eat enough for any number of reasons, ranging from reflux to chronic ear infections. While in many such children a cause can be identified, there are others where, after a thorough evaluation, everything checks out fine.

What leads some children to lack the appropriate drive to eat isn't clear. There may be poorly understood variations in brain chemistry that influence appetite and metabolism. In some cases these are normal children where the struggles over food have led to a severely dysfunctional feeding relationship. In either case the otherwise normal child who won't eat and won't grow represents a frustration for parents and pediatricians alike.

**When Size Matters: Portion Size and
How it Affects What Preschoolers Eat**

In a world where all-you-can-eat and super-size portions drive competition in the restaurant industry, what role does portion size play in how much kids eat? According to a recent study at Penn State University, it appears to depend on how old a child is. When three- and five-year-olds were provided with various servings of different sizes, the five-year-olds ate quantities in proportion to what they were served while the three-year-olds were unaffected by the size of their meal. Why is this? Younger children probably do a better job of listening to their bodies and eating what they need. Older children, on the other hand, may have learned to feed based on certain cues, such as the time of day, social context, and the size of a meal. This may, in part, explain our ongoing conflict with toddlers whose drive to eat is based more on what they need rather than what we think they need.

Fact or Fiction: Kids Shouldn't Snack

Fiction. Toddlers have tiny stomachs and can eat only so much at a sitting. Because of that, they're dependent on a little something in between their three squares. While snacks are sometimes considered the antithesis of healthy, balanced eating, they actually provide toddlers with the opportunity to round out their day with variety and extra calories.

Consider the following rules to help keep snack time healthy:

- *Choose nutritious foods.* Snack time doesn't necessarily mean junk food time. View snacks as an opportunity to provide fruits or other nutritious foods that may not be taken during meals.
- *Create patterns.* Offer similar snacks at a similar time to create consistency and structure. For example, provide a fixed number of cheese cubes or diced strawberries in a sandwich bag with a couple of ounces of diluted juice every day after nap.
- *No grazing.* Snack time, like meals, should have a beginning and an end. If snack is refused, put it away and don't offer anything until the next meal. No whining, begging, or panhandling in between.
- *Limit snacks.* No toddler should need more than two snacks a day. If you're offering three snacks a day, it will likely affect his eating at meals. If you need to give something extra in the evening, try a cup of milk.

What you've described with your child's sudden turnaround at preschool is a common phenomenon. It would appear from stories like this that the experience of socialization has a powerful influence on how children view eating. The likely key to this turnaround is that children at this age begin to see food in its larger social context. They learn that the benefits of eating begin to go beyond simply filling one's tummy and meeting basic metabolic needs. While in some cases the influence of social cues and other external factors can have a negative influence on how children eat, in cases like this it has the power to readjust a child's view of feeding to be more appropriate. In all likelihood, your child's early feeding behavior wasn't the result of anything you did or didn't do, although you may never know.

My four-year-old choked a week ago on a tortilla chip. Since that time he has refused most foods although he is drinking well and

eating soft foods like yogurt. He has lost two pounds over the course of the week, and we're concerned. What's going on?

This is probably best described as a transient feeding aversion, and it's actually quite common. When children have a frightening choking experience, they sometimes develop a panic response the next time they are faced with chewing and swallowing anything but the softest foods. Interestingly, some children will be fine for a few days after the initial choking event then suddenly develop this problem.

Unfortunately, there is no defined therapy for this problem and if left to its own it usually resolves within three to four weeks. It's critical that you allow your child to eat on his own terms during this period of crisis. Soft foods like yogurt, ice cream, and blended beverages often do the trick. Any efforts at forcing solids in this situation will only prolong the problem and compound the anxiety felt by the child. Be sure to have your son evaluated by your physician. In unusual cases where the aversion is slow to improve, a behavior modification psychologist may be helpful in reversing this pattern of fear.

My four-year-old often complains of bellyache after eating. Could he be allergic to something he's eating? Is it possible he just doesn't want to eat?

Allergies have to be one of the first concerns expressed by parents when their child experiences pain after meals. But as simple an explanation as it may sound, allergy is rarely the cause of isolated bellyache. Children experiencing food allergy at this age typically will have other symptoms, such as hives, wheezing, or congestion. Oftentimes there will be some history of significant allergic reaction to one of the common allergens (nuts, fish, milk, soy) before this age. A more likely explanation for your child's bellyache is constipation or dyspepsia.

Dyspepsia is a general medical word describing acid-related symptoms from heartburn, ulcer, or gastritis. Gastritis is a condition describing irritation of the lining of the stomach. It occurs most commonly after a viral infection and can last for weeks before resolving on its own. Gastritis occasionally can be caused by a bacterial infection in the stomach. While ulcers can occur in children, they are less common than gastritis and are much shorter lived than those seen in adults. When children experience reflux (or heartburn), it is often associated with irritation of the stomach.

Constipation is usually suspected when children make remarkably few trips to the toilet or, on the other hand, make frequent, brief trips throughout the day. Children can become so full of stool that they lose the sensation of when something is there and lack the "drive" to use the toilet. Sometimes that persistent sense of fullness can lead to a recurrent urge to go that may not be relieved despite numerous trips to the potty. In either case, children will often complain of pain after eating or interrupt meals with cramping because the colon squeezes when the stomach begins to fill.

While it's OK to look for these problems, be sure to talk to your doctor before self-diagnosing and treating anything. A number of problems can lead kids to hurt while eating, and the listed ones represent only a couple of the most common ones. Your doctor may choose to have your child undergo specific tests to pinpoint the problem before tailoring a treatment program specific to your child's age and medical needs.

With regard to the possibility that he just isn't interested in eating, this is easily exposed by presenting a more appealing option, such as dessert. If his pain is precipitated by vegetables and relieved with a banana split, you have your answer.

JUICE JUNKIES

How important is juice to a toddler's diet?

Juice has no importance in a toddler's diet. Despite the fact that they're fortified with some of the more popular vitamins, juices lessen a toddler's fragile appetite and can lead to a decrease in eating healthier foods. Juice should be regarded as a treat that complements a toddler's balanced diet.

I've always been told that a child's juice should be diluted. Is there any truth to this, and when is it OK to give a child full-strength juice?

Considering that juice should represent only a small part of any child's diet, it shouldn't matter how you prepare it. The addition of water to juice remains, however, a common practice among parents and pediatricians like myself. It's unclear where the dilution of juice had its beginnings, although it would appear to arise from the understanding that juice represents a dietary extra with the potential to erode a child's fragile appetite. If you limit your child's juice consumption to ten ounces (four to six ounces for children between six to twelve months) a day, dilution is unlikely to make a difference at any age. If, however, you find that you've created a juice junkie, dilution may be a way to limit your child's exposure to the "empty" calories that juice provides.

My pediatrician says that my daughter drinks too much juice. I have offered her alternatives but she refuses to drink anything else. What should I do?

You've created a juice junkie. Don't worry, you're not alone. Many parents find themselves with children who have

---

First Impressions Count

Kids establish an *eating pattern imprint* around the age of five to seven years much as they establish a body image during preadolescence. And once the imprint is made, it is difficult to change. Kids imprint how foods should be prepared (fried or baked) and how meals should be eaten (at the table or in front of the TV). Scrambled eggs for breakfast but never for dinner? Gotta have dessert even if I'm full! This is what your imprint is telling you. And it's these feeding patterns that you facilitate early on that create your child's impression of what, when, and how to eat as adults.

come to use juice as a pacifier. Offering a juice box to a rambunctious toddler may keep the peace when out in public but it's shortsighted and may lead to the exclusion of other more healthful alternatives, such as milk or water.

In this case of a child who refuses to take anything but juice, a gradual program is likely to work best. Begin by offering water or milk once a day in place of juice. Another approach is to dilute the child's juice with one part water to one part juice. This can gradually be decreased to one-quarter juice, three-quarters water, and so on. Remember that juice doesn't need to be eliminated completely. It can be reserved as a treat and limited to ten ounces per day. As long as water is the only alternative for the child, she'll drink it if she's thirsty. There's yet to be a case of a child who became dehydrated over limited access to juice.

Juice and Failure to Thrive

As innocent and nutritious as juice appears, excessive intake has been suspected to cause poor growth in children. The research on the juice-growth association is controversial. Studies have shown an association between excessive juice intake and everything from failure to thrive to obesity and stunting. Other studies (supported by the baby food industry) have been published that refute the common belief that juice may not be the best thing for kids.

So what's a parent to do? Common sense and an understanding that all things are OK in moderation probably will serve you best. Independent of what any study says, anyone who's ever lived with a toddler knows that after polishing off an eight-ounce bottle of juice, his appetite for more nutritious alternatives is likely to be attenuated. While a couple of bottles of juice at snack time are unlikely to affect your child's ultimate height and weight, anything more than that, over time, could impact her growth rate. When you hear begging for juice, use common sense and understand that your toddler can't.

Does juice give children diarrhea?

Juice can give children diarrhea when drunk in excess. When the amount of sugar in a child's small intestine exceeds what it's capable of digesting and absorbing, it spills into the colon, where it creates diarrhea. Some juices, such as apple, pear, and prune juice, contain significant amounts of sorbitol, which is a nonabsorbable sugar. When these juices are consumed in anything more than modest amounts, diarrhea is inevitable.

Is white grape juice healthier than other juices for children?

When talking about any kind of juice, "healthy" is a relative term. White grape juice has received attention in the press due to research done in the mid-1990s that demonstrated less spillage of sugar into the colon when compared with apple juice. It's this excess sugar in the colon that leads to the diarrhea typically associated with excess juice intake.

> **How Much Should Your Toddler Be Drinking?**
>
> Children need between eight and twelve cups of liquid per day. Milk, 100 percent juice, and the liquid in food all contribute to a child's fluid needs. Don't worry about counting ounces; most children will drink according to how much fluid they need. They're pretty good at self-regulating.

The next question becomes "What does this mean for the average toddler?" Probably not much, assuming that juice plays a balanced role in your child's diet. When drunk in volumes of ten ounces or less per day, all forms of juice should be equally well tolerated and no one juice should be considered more healthful than another.

THE SPITTING TODDLER

I've heard that reflux should be gone by a year. My eighteen-month-old was diagnosed with reflux as an infant, and he still spits up once every other day. Should I be concerned?

Most cases of infant reflux resolve between the ages of four and twelve months. By that time a baby's digestive system has matured to the point that the tummy empties efficiently. Vertical posture along with the advancement of a solid diet also help the spitting infant to get well. Once beyond a year, there's a chance that he has something a little more involved than garden-variety spitting. Unusual forms of inflammation in the upper intestine can cause an occasional vomit. Partial

---

**Fact or Fiction: The Use of Cranberry Juice Lowers the Risk
of Urinary Tract Infection**

Fact. Cranberries contain compounds (proanthocyanidins) that have been found to prevent certain types of bacteria from sticking to the wall of the bladder. It's this sticking activity by bacteria that allow them to take hold and multiply in the urinary system.

So does this mean that you should be giving cranberry juice to your toddler to prevent urinary tract infections (UTIs)? Not necessarily, although studies support the role of cranberry juice in the prevention of UTIs in children with spina bifida. Be sure to talk to your doctor. If your toddler is having frequent urinary infections, it most likely represents a larger problem than something a little juice can fix.

---

blockage of the upper intestine due to a subtle developmental defect can show in just this way. Even basic reflux that's gone on longer than usual can lead to irritation of the esophagus (swallowing tube), warranting further evaluation.

While you should definitely be concerned about your toddler's persistent vomiting, most causes are easily fixed with medication. It's unlikely that an operation will be necessary. Your son probably should be evaluated by a pediatric gastroenterologist, and his evaluation will likely include an X-ray study of the upper intestine and possibly an upper endoscopy. Until then, hold off on steam cleaning the carpets.

Judging a Juice by Its Cover

While we tend to think of juice as a healthy alternative for our children, a closer look at the label shows that there may be less juice and nutrition than what meets the eye. Look for labels that state *100% juice*. This indicates that what you're buying is the real thing. The terms "drinks," "cocktails," "beverages," and "punches" indicate that the juice in that particular product has been diluted. Look at the fine print to see how much you're actually getting.

Remember that "natural" is in the eye of the beholder (or the juice manufacturer), and that the law regulating the use of this attractive term is loose when it comes to labeling. Corn syrup, one of the favored sweeteners, is considered natural.

My baby is fifteen months old and, once or twice a week, throws up undigested food hours after he has eaten it. Is this behavioral?

It's very unlikely that your son's vomiting is behavioral. The fact that he's throwing up old food suggests that he's having a hard time emptying food from his stomach. This is referred to as *gastroparesis*, and it may represent nothing more than a poor squeezing mechanism in the stomach (in the old days referred to as a weak stomach). Gastroparesis may come about from irritation in the stomach or upper intestine that's preventing the normal squeezing of the stomach. Some children can develop gastroparesis after a bad viral gastroenteritis. Most cases go away on their own although it can take weeks to months to resolve completely. This should be evaluated by your physician and a pediatric gastroenterologist.

My three-year-old has learned to make himself throw up when he's upset. Is this harmful and what's the best way to handle it?

Any sort of dramatic behavior like this is usually learned and reinforced by your reaction. Sometimes toddlers will pull this one out of their back pocket when they want to divert attention away from something bad that they've been up to. Other times it may be used to draw attention to their situation when they feel that they've not been given the attention they deserve. As hard as it may be, the best way to handle this sort of obnoxious behavior is to ignore it. The more attention drawn to it and the greater the reaction on your part, the more likely the behavior is to be perpetuated.

Assuming that this isn't a problem that hangs on for more than a few months, it shouldn't be harmful. Chronic vomiting can lead to irritation and burning of the swallowing tube. If the vomiting is occurring at times other than when he's upset, be sure to have it checked out.

WATCHING OUT FOR NUMBER TWO

My eighteen-month-old passes whole vegetables in his diaper. Does this mean that he's not digesting them?

Vegetables in the diaper are fairly common at this age, and it's no cause for alarm. Intestinal transit time, or the time it takes food to get from top to bottom, is faster in toddlers, and the result is occasional undigested food in the diaper. In most cases parents report vegetables since the fiber found in vegetables takes more time to break down. Don't worry about losing nutrients. A child's body will take what it needs, and these occasional veggies represent only a small fraction of what your child is taking in.

My two-year-old is beginning to strain with bowel movements. Is this a diet problem?

While diet is infrequently the sole cause of a child's pooping difficulties, it certainly can play the role of accomplice. The diet items that can lead to problems most commonly include excessive milk, cheese, and dairy products. These are considered low-residue foods that form sticky, claylike stools that are difficult to pass. Fluid is also a key dietary factor in producing poops that are soft and painless to pass. Fiber certainly tends to help matters but it is highly overrated in toddlers . . . that is, when you can get them to take foods with significant fiber.

Some children, despite a model diet, have a difficult time for reasons that are hard to put a finger on. Just as children differ in their size, shape, and personality, so too do they differ in the way their colon works. As the organ responsible for the absorption of excess fluid from digestive material, the efficiency of the colon may differ from child to child. The motility, or squeezing action, of the colon also may be different in your child. So some of what we experience with constipated children goes well beyond diet and gets into physiology and variations of normal.

Medically Speaking: Toddler's Diarrhea

If mood instability and emerging independence weren't enough to deal with in your eighteen-month-old, the idea of chronic diarrhea is usually more than most parents can handle. One of the most common causes of chronic diarrhea in this age group is a condition referred to as *toddler's diarrhea*. This is a poorly understood condition where children have several watery, gasless, painless stools per day. These are often marked by the presence of undigested food in the diarrhea. Typically children with toddler's diarrhea are happy, healthy, and unaffected by their runny poop. In fact, most pediatric gastroenterologists consider this diagnosis when the diarrhea bothers the parents more than it does the child.

The cause of toddler's diarrhea is not well understood although it is felt to represent a condition where the intestines move their contents through faster than normal. Some experts feel that this problem is initiated by a viral infection. Others suspect that toddler's diarrhea represents a temporary problem of intestinal motility limited to this age group. While the cause may be unclear, it's an entirely benign condition that can last up to several months.

There are very few effective therapies for this problem, although some children respond to the addition of a supplemental fiber source. Some children respond to treatment with a particular antibiotic, but the effect is often short-lived.

In children who don't respond to the most basic recommendations of increasing fluids, limiting milk, and improving fiber, medical help is usually necessary. This is particularly important in the two-year-old since, as we approach toilet training, we like to assure that pooping is a pleasant experience. If it ain't pleasant in the diaper, there's no way it's going to be pleasant as we transition to the potty.

In these cases most pediatricians and pediatric gastroenterologists use stool softeners like milk of magnesia or mineral oil. These are nonhabit-forming preparations that soften stools and allow the child to pass stool with less effort. And passing stools with less effort is the key here. Once children at this age learn that pooping is associated with pain, they'll do everything in their power to avoid it. These children are referred to as *stool withholders*, and they can be challenging to turn around once they've started. If you think your child may be in this category, see your pediatrician. Waiting never fixes this problem and may ultimately make matters worse for her . . . and you.

How much fiber should a two-year-old get?

Fiber is a bit of a double-edged sword in kids. While it helps maintain bowel regularity, it also can take away an appetite. Remember that while we all tend to think wonderful things about fiber, it really does nothing to help children grow and, in effect, has no nutritional value. This is of particular importance with the picky eater where every bite needs to pack as many calories as possible. Don't worry too much about fiber. There are other issues of greater importance in this age group, such as actually getting them to eat. Offer your child a variety of fruit and vegetable finger selections, and over the course of a day, he's likely to get all he needs.

Is low-fat or skim milk less constipating than whole milk?

No. The constipating nature of excessive milk intake occurs independent of what kind of milk it is. If your toddler is having a hard time with her stools, try limiting her milk intake to twelve to fifteen ounces per day. If your child has had difficulties with her growth, be sure to discuss this with your pediatrician since milk may represent a significant source of her calories and protein.

Sources of Natural Fiber

What your child will eat will vary from day to day and week to week. In general, try to keep the focus on an appealing assortment of fruits, vegetables, and grains and consider the following fiber suggestions:

Wheat germ—add to yogurt or ice cream

Strawberries and bananas—add to cereal

Pears and apples—serve with the peel to increase fiber

Applesauce—add to the top of a waffle or pancake

Peas, lentils, and kidney beans—use in casseroles and other dishes

Minced carrot, zucchini, or squash—use with spaghetti sauce instead of ground beef

Whole wheat bread—use instead of white. Look for "whole wheat flour," not enriched wheat

Dried fruits such as apricots and raisins

Sweet potatoes—serve diced or mashed

I've heard that milk can damage the lining of the bowel. How do I know if this is occurring in my child?

When we speak about milk causing injury to the lining of a baby's intestine, we're usually referring to the child under a year. The lining of the infant's intestine is particularly sensitive to the type of protein found in milk out of the carton. This is why it's recommended that milk be withheld until a child's first birthday. How is a cow's-milk-based formula different from this? The protein in standard formula does come from cows, just like the milk out of the carton, but it is heated to be less reactive and it's added in much smaller quantities than that found in regular cow's milk.

You Shouldn't Need a Calculator to Feed Your Child

You may read that your child's daily fiber intake in grams should be equal to his age plus five. While it may be true, predicting a toddler's intake from day to day and knowing what grams are going in with particular meals requires a degree of preoccupation on your part that isn't healthy. Provide your child with a variety of nutritious, fiber-containing foods and avoid feeding plans that involve the use of a calculator.

Assuming that a baby has had an uneventful infancy, she should be able to tolerate cow's milk without any difficulty after a year. In rare cases, if milk is taken in very large quantities (greater than thirty to forty ounces per day), a toddler may experience some irritation in the colon marked by diarrhea, cramping with stools, and occasionally visible blood. In the absence of these symptoms, your pediatrician may be able to test your child's stool for the presence of microscopic blood, which may be the only indication of a problem.

My toddler's stool is sometimes bright green. What does this mean?

As dramatic as it may appear, it means nothing. Stool starts green due to the presence of bile that is dumped into the intestine way up near the stomach. During its fantastic journey it gradually turns the brown color typically associated with stool. Some toddlers will have rapid transit of food through the intestine and their diaper will show more green than brown. In most cases this is a variant of normal. It also can be seen after or during a viral gastrointestinal infection. In this case the electric green stool should be short-lived.

Why does apple juice give some children gas?

Apple juice, like pear and prune juice, contains a nonabsorbable sugar called *sorbitol*. Depending on the bacteria

---

Tots Who Toot

Gas in toddlers is often as much a social issue as a medical issue, given their natural disregard for proper social conduct. For those of us who spend a lot of time thinking about gas, we tend to put tootin' toddlers into one of a couple of categories:

- *Air swallowing.* This is one of the most common causes of excessive intestinal gas in children. Basically air that's swallowed needs to be belched or otherwise endure the fantastic journey through the intestinal system. Or, in other words, what doesn't come up must go down. The most common causes of air swallowing are excessive thumb sucking, pacifier use, crying, or chronic mouth breathing due to sinus congestion.

- *Poor absorption of sugars.* Sugars that aren't absorbed properly in the upper intestine are usually fermented in the large intestine, and gas is the result. This is very common after viral infections when the lining of the small intestine isn't up to snuff. But beyond a couple of weeks after a stomach bug, it's very unusual that the small intestine doesn't do what it's supposed to. If, however, a child exceeds her capacity to naturally absorb sugar through the excessive intake of juice, gas is a predictable outcome. Juice, sports drinks, and other sugary beverages should be limited to ten ounces per day.

Does the odor of a child's gas indicate what may be going on? Usually not. More than likely the odor represents the mixture of gases produced by the bacteria that inhabit your child's colon. This is also influenced by constituents of her diet and what's being fed to the colon. The foul-smelling, "rotten-egg" gas that some children pass means that your child is one of the chosen few members of the population harboring methane-producing bacteria in the colon. While it isn't dangerous to the child, it may seem that way for those who have to live with her. If your child's gas doesn't appear to be a postviral phenomenon, or an excess sugar or air-swallowing problem, consider a two-week course of acidophilus (active yeast culture) to adjust the bacterial flora in the colon.

---

that happen to inhabit your child's colon, it can be fermented to a greater or lesser degree, resulting in gas. Most children experience no problems with diarrhea or gas when their juice intake is limited to ten ounces a day.

SPOONS, CUPS, AND CHAIRS

At what age should a child stop using a high chair?

There are no rules about the duration of high chair use, and it's fine to use as long as it fits her rapidly growing behind. Most children are able to make the move from high chair to booster seat between their second and third birthday or whenever feeding begins to become more contained. Since spills and smears take on a new dimension at the table, you'll want to make sure she has a basic understanding of what kind of behavior is accepted and what isn't.

When does a child begin using a fork or spoon?

It depends on your definition of "use." A child should be offered a spoon beginning around twelve months. At this age, she will use the spoon to haphazardly move food from the bowl to her high chair and from her high chair to her bib. It won't be until fourteen to eighteen months that a child will gradually begin to hone her motor skills and be able to use a spoon for a purpose more closely approximating its intended function. By two years a child should be able to use a spoon with moderate spillage and have it down by three years. Remember that babies need short, easy-to-grasp utensils, which are very different from what you may have used to feed with initially.

When starting out, prepare the spoon with samples of food since the skill of scooping food from the bowl will come later than the skill of lifting it from the bowl to the mouth. Left on their own, children will figure this out, but a little help never hurt.

Skilled and proficient use of a fork isn't achieved until closer to three years of age. Be patient early on. While messy, the trial-and-error disasters of utensil-feeding in early toddlerhood are essential to mastering this skill.

At what age can a child cut with a knife?

You've got a bit of a wait. Children will normally begin to use a knife for cutting at around eight years of age. A knife can be used for spreading around five years of age.

When should a child stop using a bottle?

Most pediatricians advocate abandoning the bottle between twelve and fifteen months. What's wrong with the continued use of a bottle? Nothing, really, except that beginning late in the first year, children develop the ability to drink from a tippy cup. This is a more developmentally appropriate way to feed your toddler, and it should be your goal. There is no good reason to keep your child on a bottle unless, of course, she is in complete control of you and your household. In this case you have problems ahead of you bigger than a stubborn bottle habit.

My sixteen-month-old won't drink from a cup. I haven't forced the issue because I'm afraid if I don't give him his bottle, he'll become dehydrated or stop eating. What should I do?

Concern over dehydration is a common obstacle to getting children to give up their bottles. While it may seem that your child is taking in only minimal amounts of fluid during the transition, there has yet to be a documented case of a child who became dehydrated coming off of the bottle. Given the option of thirst or a cup, a toddler ultimately will choose the cup.

You may try a transition lid, which fits on the top of a traditional bottle and has a spout shorter than the typical tippy cup. This compromise may be easier for your child to take, and he may need more time. Consider taking your child to the local baby superstore to choose a cup on his own. The novelty of a color and shape chosen personally may make all the difference.

My fifteen-month-old son will take only juice out of a tippy cup and still insists on a bottle for his milk. What do I do?

As tough as the situation may seem, the solution is simple: Drop the bottle and make milk the only option with meals. It also helps to have his milk cup at the high chair before sitting down and to keep all bottles out of sight. Continue to offer water or juice during the day (limit juice to approximately ten ounces) with snacks. Be sure to stay true to the idea that when milk is offered, it's the only option. Most children will turn the corner within a couple of weeks but not without some protest. Remember that children will drink milk out of a tippy cup before they go thirsty.

For the occasional child who is a poor eater and still refuses milk from the tippy cup despite a firm, consistent approach, flavored milk may do the trick. To a child like this, milk is an important source of nutrition, and it's reasonable to do whatever it takes to maintain appropriate intake of the protein and fat that it offers. Most major dairies market chocolate-, vanilla-, peach- and banana-flavored whole and low-fat milk. As with all toddlers, choose whole milk. If the idea of flavored milk doesn't settle well with you, consider starting with this and slowly mixing in plain milk week by week.

If your child has had problems gaining weight and won't take milk despite your best efforts, talk to your pediatrician. He may need a more formal assessment by a pediatric dietician who is in a position to recommend alternatives and tricks to help maintain an appropriate diet.

When should a child make the transition from a tippy cup to a regular cup?

The big question here is not when she can use a regular cup but when she is proficient enough with it to use it as her regular source of drinking. Most children can begin using a regular cup at around twenty-four months, but it isn't until three years or older that they begin to do it with any proficiency. As a means of exhibiting their ever-growing need for independence, many kids will initiate this step by asking to have their cup lid removed or not attached in the first place. Remember to offer very little liquid in the cup at first and to have plenty of towels on hand. How much of a mess you're willing to put up with may dictate when you begin to use a regular cup full time.

My eighteen-month-old screams, arches, and throws a fit whenever she's put into the high chair. Why is this?

At first glance this isn't good. It suggests that your child is somehow fearful of what's about to happen, perhaps because of what's gone on in the past. So the first issue to consider is what's gone on in the past to initiate this sort of behavior. What is it that's led her to think such horrible things about the feeding experience? Are you overbearing with the spoon? Are you force-feeding your child because of your own frustration? Have you crossed the division of responsibility that dictates our feeding role as parents? Consider the possibility that this is a bib issue. Some toddlers freak out at the idea of a bib around their neck, although this problem is typically quite obvious. Have you considered taking off the high chair tray and pulling the chair right up to the table?

The answer to these questions can come only when you've been honest with yourself about the feeding experience you've provided for your daughter. While your intentions may be good, any pressure that you provide during mealtime will ultimately backfire, and that may be the case here.

As far as what to do at this point, it's clear that the high chair is where she needs to eat. Removing her at this time would only avoid the issue and put you in the habit of feeding her somewhere less appropriate. Read the other questions in this section and try to gain a clearer understanding of what's normal for children this age. More important, try to understand how you may be reacting to her normal behavior and let her do her own thing. Any changes you make today will take days to weeks to turn around because of what she's learned about feeding. Keep her in the high chair, let her arch, provide her with an appealing variety of tasty finger foods, and let her do what she will. In time this will pass.

My toddler will eat only while sitting on my lap. What do I do?
The first question is, how did she get in your lap to begin with? As discussed, a toddler's mealtime routine needs firm limits that you establish and maintain from early on. Once a child has the option to be coddled in your arms during mealtime, she'll always choose that over the cold, lonely confines of the high chair. Just like a bottle or pacifier that's been around a little too long, breaking these habits can be difficult. Your only option here is to put her in the high chair and let her cry. This may go on for two to three days, but don't give in. Remember that mealtime has a beginning and an end—if she chooses to cry rather than eat, don't make the mistake of offering dinner an hour after dinner is over. Just think how excited she'll be to see breakfast . . . in her high chair.

When can a child begin to use a straw?
Most children can begin to get the knack of a straw down between eighteen and twenty-four months. Expect bubbles, backwash, and sputtering at first, and don't be surprised if the novelty of the straw leads to a transient obsession. You can put this to work by introducing drinks through the straw that may have been refused in the past.

When can a child be allowed to chew gum?
Gum chewing should be considered an occasional treat and not a developmental feeding milestone. Should you choose to offer your child gum, wait until close to four years old, when the risk of choking will be minimized. Use sugar-free gum and don't allow its use during exercise or play.

Chapter 1

Special Concerns

Beyond the basics of starting solids and warming formula, other nutrition questions and situations will come up once your child grows beyond toddlerhood. Many relate to the overconsumption or underconsumption of food; others involve vitamins, food additives, and other things children may need or not need. Ultimately the classic preoccupation of the young parent, getting the child to eat, is replaced by thoughts of whether she's eating right.

Once past the toddler years, your involvement and concern should evolve to focus on healthful, balanced choices that will set the pace for future eating habits. You need to be more aware of what your kids are eating and how it fits into a healthy lifestyle of exercise and other activities. Your concerns now should be different from when you started your child on table food.

One of the concerns of parents is the way their child looks. Is she too fat or too thin, and is the way she looks any indication of how she'll look as an adult? While your child's weight shouldn't be a preoccupation, it should be a health issue followed and addressed no differently from dental care or immunizations. But unlike dental concerns and the diseases we so compulsively immunize for, obesity is on the rise among children. Most experts agree that this is a consequence of a sedentary lifestyle and a high-fat diet. While it's easy to call this a social problem, it's more likely a parent problem. Children learn what they live, and a sensible diet and lifestyle is the responsibility of every parent. When it comes to weight and dietary lifestyle issues with children, it's definitely a case where an ounce of prevention is far easier than a pound of cure.

NUTRITION AND THE SICK CHILD

How much should a child be drinking when he has a stomach virus?

Keeping your child hydrated is one of the most immediate concerns when she's got a stomach illness. The issue of hydration is what brings children to the emergency room for evaluation most often, so if you can keep your child from getting to that point, you can save everyone a lot of headache. The bottom line is that you've got to keep up with whatever your child is losing through diarrhea or throwing up. It's impossible to estimate how much that is since illnesses vary as much as children do. Give her as much as she'll take and watch for wet diapers. For a vomiting illness, this is best done with small quantities of rehydration solution or diluted juice. Some children will vomit after drinking anything over half an ounce, and these kids will need to be fed by a teaspoon at a time. Watch for dry mouth (and an inability to make bubbles), sunken eyes, lethargy, and a decrease in wet diapers. By the time you get to this point, you'll need to consider more detailed advice from your pediatrician or a visit to the local ER.

Why do pediatricians sometimes recommend giving babies half-strength formula when they're sick with a stomach flu?

To understand the reasoning behind the half-strength recommendation, it's important to understand a little about normal sugar absorption and intestinal viral infections. The lining of the upper small intestine contains enzymes that are involved in the digestion and absorption of the different sugars in our diet. Under normal circumstances, sugars are absorbed and effectively removed from our food high in the small intestine by these important enzymes. Gastrointestinal viruses interfere

---

Fact or Fiction: Starve a Cold, Feed a Fever

Fiction. There's no evidence that the outcome of colds or fever have anything to do with how much or how little children are fed. Let them eat cake . . . or chicken soup.

---

with the normal process of digestion by attacking the intestinal lining and temporarily destroying some of these enzymes.

When sugars are ingested by a child suffering from such a virus, they are not absorbed properly and make their way into the large intestine, the part of our digestive system inhabited by large numbers of bacteria. The bacteria that inhabit the colon are more than happy to take care of the misdirected sugars through fermentation. The result is gas, diarrhea, and stomach growling—all trademarks of the typical childhood intestinal infection.

Enter the half-strength formula. By offering a child formula that is diluted or cut in half, she is receiving half of the normal amount of sugar. Since half as much sugar is making its way to the large intestine, the child experiences less diarrhea, cramping, and pain. Sometimes a child's diarrhea is so bad that the intestines tolerate very little sugar. Under these circumstances, children usually require bowel rest, where nothing is given by mouth and the child's fluid needs are met intravenously.

Under normal circumstances, a gastrointestinal viral infection lasts for only a few days. Unfortunately, the damage left behind by most viruses lasts longer. It can take up to a week after the virus is gone before the intestinal lining is healed and the body has regenerated its important enzymes. Even then a child's bowel pattern may not come back to normal for some weeks since the motility or squeezing rhythm of the bowel is often thrown off by a stomach infection.

Remember that half-strength formula is also half-calorie and half-protein formula. It contains half of everything a child needs for normal growth and development. As a result, reduced-strength formulas shouldn't be used for more than two or three days unless directed by your pediatrician.

What is it about oral rehydration solutions that make them better for sick children than juices or soda?

What makes oral rehydration solutions like Pedialyte® and Rehydralyte® special is their balance of sugar and salts. It's known that when sugar and salt are present in proper proportion, their absorption helps facilitate the absorption of water. In children who are extremely dehydrated, plain water or juice without the proper balance of minerals can lead to a dangerous condition called water intoxication. Sodas and fruit juices contain such high sugar levels that they may even *contribute* to a child's diarrhea when drunk in excess.

The truth is, however, that most cases of viral diarrhea contracted by typical well-nourished American children are mild in comparison to those that rehydration solution are really designed for. For generations flat ginger ale and homemade juice concoctions have been used with success to treat the mild and transient cases of diarrhea that children frequently encounter. If it's anything more than a mild case of the squirts, talk to your doctor. Otherwise use what it takes to keep the diapers wet and the lips moist.

Don't Make Formula with Rehydration Solution

When preparing a child's concentrated or powdered formula, be sure to use water and not rehydration solutions. Using the latter can lead to dangerously excessive levels of certain minerals.

Does oral rehydration solution contain the same calories as formula?

While oral rehydration solution allows a smooth transition from sick tummy to normal feeding, it lacks the nutritional value of breast milk or formula. Rehydration solution contains no protein and only three calories per ounce. This is about fifteen percent of the calories found in standard infant formula.

Is flavored rehydration solution OK for young babies?

Despite the fact that most babies aren't going to be able to discriminate fruity-fruit from bubble gum, flavored rehydration solutions are perfectly safe for use in babies.

What is a BRAT diet?

Despite your fantasy that there may be a diet to control your child's mischievous ways, this is nothing more than an old-fashioned protocol for diarrhea. Consisting of bananas, rice, applesauce, and toast, this old standby was felt to be more binding for children with recovering viral gastroenteritis. While the BRAT diet is unlikely to do any harm, it's more apt to keep demanding parents busy while their child's body recovers on its own.

My fourteen-month-old recently got over a bad cold, and she now refuses to drink milk. Why is this, and is there anything I can do about it?

Sometimes a severe upper respiratory infection will change the way children taste food, and it may temporarily turn them off to certain things. This is usually a temporary problem but one that can last up to a few weeks. Before setting an ultimatum about her milk, give her a week without it, allowing her to substitute with diluted juice and water. When you reintroduce it, serve it only with meals and offer nothing else to drink should she refuse it. If this is refused and you're dumping cup after cup over the period of a few days, try the option of a flavored milk, such as vanilla or strawberry. The novelty or change may be enough to do the trick. If the idea of flavored milk leaves you sour, you can slowly dilute it with regular milk so that you ultimately transition her back to the regular stuff over a couple of weeks.

If your child is taking her milk from a bottle, another option would be to try to introduce a tippy cup at this point. Again, the novelty of a new appliance may be enough to make her forget about her distaste for milk, and it could make for an easy transition off the bottle.

Our two-year-old has had diarrhea for the past three to four weeks. The pediatrician told us that it was a virus, but he continues to have diarrhea. We have kept him off of milk and offered juice to keep him hydrated. Is there anything else we can do?

As frustrating as ongoing diarrhea may be, sometimes our attempts to help it are often part of the problem. It's not uncommon that parents push juices and avoid milk in order to prevent dehydration. This excessive use of juice is often the source of ongoing diarrhea in the child with a recovering viral illness. Especially when the lining of the intestine has been injured by a virus, the amount of sugar tolerated by a child may be limited. And what's not absorbed in the upper intestine makes its way into the colon, where the result is diarrhea. Be sure to limit your child's intake of juice and sports drinks to ten ounces a day to avoid this common scenario.

Fact or Fiction: If Your Child Has a Cold, He Should Avoid Drinking Milk

Probably fiction. The use of milk in children with gastroenteritis is a source of long-standing debate. While a severe intestinal infection is likely to cause some loss of lactase, the enzyme responsible for digesting the milk sugar lactose, most infections aren't that severe and the majority of children are able to tolerate milk just fine. While a day or two off of milk or formula isn't likely to cause your child any harm, remember that this is the primary source of protein and calories for infants and young toddlers. Any break from good nutrition more than forty-eight hours long is likely to represent a significant compromise in your child's nutrition and ultimately in her ability to recover.

Should temporary intolerance of lactose represent a serious concern to you or your pediatrician, infants can be placed on a lactose-free infant formula temporarily. Most soy-based toddler formulas contain no lactose and can be used until everyone's satisfied with the idea that the worst is over (usually two weeks).

THE CHILD WHO WON'T GROW

What is failure to thrive?

Children who consistently fail to gain weight at a normal rate are characterized as having failure to thrive, or FTT. Its definition has less to do with a child's weight at any one point in time than it does with a child's weight gain over a period of time. For example, a child who grows along the tenth percentile through the first year may be considered smaller than

90 percent of one-year-olds but shouldn't raise concern that anything's wrong. On the other hand, a child who grows at the seventy-fifth percentile through seven months of age and then fails to gain any weight for the last five months of her first year would be considered to have failure to thrive. While both babies may wind up at the same weight at a year, the second baby's failure to gain any weight over the last five months represents a problem that needs to be evaluated. So FTT has to do with how much weight is gained *over time* rather than how much a baby weighs at any given point.

While this simple example may seem straightforward, there are plenty of exceptions and subtleties that make the interpretation of growth patterns a true art. Look to your pediatrician for guidance if you think there's a problem, and remember that a $6.50 book will never replace their experience and wisdom.

Why Children Don't Gain Weight

While a number of problems can cause children to grow poorly, most fall into one of three major categories. Identifying which category the child falls into represents the first step in identifying a specific cause.

1. Not enough calories. This represents the most common reason children fail to grow. Simply put, if a child doesn't get enough fuel, she can't build muscle and fat. A child's failure to take in adequate calories can be caused by a variety of problems, ranging from complicated reflux to chronic ear infections.

2. Poor absorption of calories. If your child eats like a horse but still can't put on weight, she may not be absorbing her calories. This is referred to as *malabsorption* and is often associated with chronic diarrhea, bloating, or oily stools.

3. Increased demand for calories. If your child eats well, absorbs all of his nutrients, but still can't hold his weight, it may mean that he needs more calories than the average child. Often children with chronic heart or lung disease require extra calories to make up for the overtime their hard-working organs are putting in. Children who need more calories are typically easy to recognize and have been identified as having a chronic disease. If your child has passed a basic physical, this is a very unlikely explanation for his poor growth.

Our child grew at the ninetieth percentile until he was thirteen months. Over the past three months he has had very little growth, placing him at the seventy-fifth percentile. Is this failure to thrive and do we need to do anything about it?

This is not FTT but more likely what's referred to as catch-down growth. During the first two years of life, babies who started off big often will go a couple of months with little growth as a way of bringing themselves back to their genetic set point. Once they're back to where they belong, they will once again resume along their normal growth curve. Assuming that your child is otherwise well, there's nothing to be done besides regular monitoring of height and weight.

Modern Curves

With the dawn of the new millennium, doctors in the United States have a whole new way to watch kids grow. The National Center for Health Statistics recently published a new set of growth curves for birth through age twenty. The current growth charts are based on new data and statistical analysis and replace the previous charts made in 1977 by the National Center for Health Statistics.

What's new with how we're looking at kids?

- The new growth curves are more representative of our country's ethnic diversity and rising interest in breast-feeding. The previous curves were based primarily on formula-fed white children from the Midwest born between 1929 and 1975.
- Children can be tracked to age twenty instead of eighteen.
- The new curves allow more detailed tracking of growth percentiles at the extremes of size above 95 percent and below 5 percent.
- Doctors can now plot a child's *body mass index* (BMI), a number that indicates whether a child's weight is proportional to her height. The BMI can help identify children who are overweight or at risk for becoming overweight as adults.

For more information, check out *www.cdc.gov/growthcharts*.

We have heard that a child's nutrition can affect his intellectual development. Our son is eighteen months old and he has always been just below the fifth percentile for weight and twenty-fifth percentile for height. Do we need to be concerned?

No. Considering that your son has grown consistently at the fifth percentile indicates that he's gaining weight at the appropriate rate. While he may be on the small side, he is nonetheless gaining weight as he should. After all, 5 percent of very normal children weigh in at the fifth percentile.

Concerning his potential for development, there's no reason to expect any problems. While nutrition can clearly affect a child's intellectual development, this usually applies to children with severe, prolonged malnutrition, such as that seen in third world countries. Keep in mind, however, that in developed countries such as the United States, specific nutrient deficiencies such as iron have been linked to suboptimal developmental in children.

Fact or Fiction: If You Double a Two-Year-Old's Height, You'll Get Her Adult Height

Fiction. Despite this commonly held wives' tale, the calculation of a child's ultimate height isn't so simple. How tall a child ultimately winds up has more to do with her parents' height than anything else. Since they are more entertaining than reliable, formulas for adult height don't play a major role in pediatric care.

If my child isn't growing, how often should his weight be checked?

This depends on your child's age, how poorly he's growing, and your pediatrician's level of concern. Breast-fed infants slow to pick up on their feeding may need daily checks while older toddlers who don't measure up may need to be followed every month or two.

If you've had thoughts of buying your own scale, consider thinking of another way to spend the money. The scales available on the typical budget are usually not accurate enough to warrant the expense and anxiety that they invariably generate. And knowing your child's weight gain or loss is useless unless you've been trained to understand what's normal and how to act on what's abnormal. Don't try this at home.

At what point does an underweight child need to be fed by tube?
Once it's clear that a child is failing to take in the calories
needed to grow, the first step is to try to find ways to get extra calories in. In babies, this can be done through the use of
more concentrated formulas that provide extra calories for
the same intake of formula. With toddlers, we can sometimes get extra calories in with the addition of rich, calorie-
dense foods such as butter, gravies, and sour cream.
Oftentimes the underweight child can be turned around with
nothing more than suggestions like these and the close per-
sonalized guidance of a pediatric dietician.

For the dangerously underweight child who fails to take
in the calories necessary for normal growth, help is often
needed through the use of a temporary feeding tube. *Feeding
tubes really serve two purposes in the underweight child.*
First, they help us prove that the child's problem is a failure
to take in calories and nothing else. In other words, if we
provide calories and a child immediately gains weight, we
know that we're probably not dealing with any type of unusual disease but rather a failure to take in the energy necessary for growth.

The second purpose of a feeding tube is, of course, to allow a child to gain weight. Through appropriate use of
nighttime supplemental feeding with a feeding pump and
occasional boluses (minimeals) of milk by day, children can
begin to show dramatic weight gain within a few weeks. Often the improved nutrition jump-starts children and stimulates their activity and appetite. Feeding tubes should be
seen as a way of resuscitating and transitioning a child back
to nutritional health. While I've never met a parent excited
about the idea of a feeding tube, I've also never met a parent
who wasn't satisfied and relieved with the end result.

Feeding tubes are about the diameter of a piece of
spaghetti and are placed through the nose and into the stomach by a nurse or physician. Some tubes can be placed and
left in for up to a month; others need more frequent replacement. In general, nasogastric feeding tubes shouldn't be

used in a child for more than two to three months since prolonged use can lead to irritation and infection of the sinuses.

I've seen canned nutritional supplements for children advertised. How do I know if my child needs one?
Madison Avenue recently has tried to convince all con-
sumers that everyone, despite their size or shape, can benefit
from the use of liquid nutritional supplements. While you
can always make the argument that it can't hurt and might

More Bang for the Buck: High-calorie Foods for Tiny Toddlers

Sometimes getting underweight toddlers to eat the amount of food necessary for
growth and catch-up can be difficult, if not impossible. One way to address this
issue is to put more calories into the things she's willing to eat. Consider the
following condiments, toppings, and snacks:

Butter (100 calories/tbsp)
- Melt and add to cereal, oatmeal, or vegetables.

Canned gravy (40 calories/tbsp)
- Pour on mashed potatoes, squash, and vegetables.

Powdered milk (33 calories/tbsp)
- Put in soups, ground beef, and casseroles for added calories and protein.

Mayonnaise (100 calories/tbsp) and sour cream (26 calories/tbsp)
- Add to potatoes; use as a dip for finger foods.

Carnation Instant Breakfast (130 calories/packet)
- Add to milk for a milkshake with extra calories and protein.

Ice cream (75 calories/ounce)
- Everyone knows what to do with this.

Peanut butter (95 calories/tbsp)
- Put on rice cakes, apples, and crackers.
- Use small amounts since this can present a choking hazard.

Cream cheese (50 calories/tbsp)
- Spread on bread, crackers, or ripe apples.

Cheese (about 100 calories/ounce)
- Grate on meats, vegetables, or casseroles.

---

help, nutritional supplements are rarely helpful to children and should be used only under the supervision of your doctor. Even among the pickiest children, liquid nutritional supplements aren't necessary unless the child demonstrates true growth failure from inadequate calories.

If a supplement is recommended for your child, you might consider supplementing whole milk with instant breakfast powder. The nutritional value is about as good, it's much less expensive, and the flavor options tend to be a lot better.

My child is sixteen months old and was placed on a nutritional supplement because she's underweight. It's supposed to be for children over a year old but she's the weight of a nine-month-old. Is this OK?
This should be fine. The concern with the use of toddler nutritional supplements in infants is the concentration and level of protein, which may be too much for small kidneys. Independent of her size, your daughter's system should be mature enough to handle a formula for toddlers.

We recently took our underweight daughter to a nutritionist for help. He wants a sample of her hair to analyze in his lab for minerals. Is this right?
No, this is wrong. As a general rule, any "nutritionist" who wants to analyze your child's hair should be assumed a quack until proven otherwise. The cases of poor growth where mineral analysis of the hair have any role in management are truly exceptional. Hair analysis does have a role in assessment of certain genetic and skin diseases as well as in the diagnosis of certain rare types of environmental poison exposure. In cases such as these, your child's care should be directly supervised by an M.D. with board certification in whatever field of medicine he claims to have expertise.

Are appetite stimulants ever used in children?
In rare and unusual circumstances, appetite stimulants are used in children. They should be used only under the supervision of a physician experienced in their use and only after

Where to Go for Help When Your Doctor May Not Be Giving You What You Need

Desperate and anxious parents frequently look for help in all of the wrong places when they think their child is in danger. And it seems there's always someone willing to lend a hand when there's money to be spent. So who are the real players in helping the nutritionally challenged child, and where do you go when you're concerned?

Pediatric Dietician

Degree: R.D. (registered dietician)
Plays a key role in the assessment of nutritional need and implementation of nutritional therapy.
Should deal exclusively or have special experience with children. Taking your underweight toddler to a dietician for adults is like bringing her to an internist for a rash—it's probably a waste of time.

Pediatric Gastroenterologist

Degree: M.D.
Most are quite accustomed to dealing with growth problems and nutritional issues especially as they relate to feeding and intestinal problems.
All pediatric gastroenterologists in the United States are trained in general pediatrics with three years of pediatric gastroenterology training after residency. Your doctor should be board certified by the American Board of Pediatrics in pediatric gastroenterology and nutrition.

Pediatric Occupational Therapist or Speech Pathologist

Degree: O.T.R. (registered occupational therapist), CCC/SLP (speech pathologist)
Pediatric occupational therapists and speech pathologists specialize in the diagnosis and management of infant and toddler feeding problems. They manage behavioral feeding aversions and treat children with special needs like a cleft palate, Down syndrome, or cerebral palsy. Like any specialist you seek for your child, they should have special training and an exclusive interest in treating children.
So how about a good old-fashioned nutritionist? Unfortunately, anyone can declare himself or herself a nutritionist without any training, education, or experience. Anyone who hands you a business card proclaiming to be a nutritionist without the proper clinical degree and qualifications should be considered a quack until proven otherwise. When in doubt, ask specifically about qualifications including education, degree, board certification, and clinical experience.

a thorough evaluation has been performed. Poor growth from poor eating can be caused by a number of diseases and conditions that may be masked with the inappropriate use of appetite stimulants.

Can vitamin supplements help increase my child's appetite?

No, vitamins do not function as appetite stimulants, and giving extra vitamins will not change a child's appetite. In unusual circumstances a vitamin or mineral deficiency can influence a person's eating through making food taste differently or affecting how the person feels. These cases are, however, extremely rare in children.

THE CHILD WHO WON'T STOP GROWING

Our six-month-old will eat just about everything and it shows. Everyone comments on how big and pudgy he is. Are we overfeeding him, and what can we do about it?

First of all, consider yourself lucky that you have a child who's healthy and gaining weight. The opposite scenario of the underweight child is much harder to fix and equally frustrating for parents.

Assuming that you're offering breast milk or formula for hunger and providing a couple of feeds a day of baby food (approximately half a jar or two tablespoons), you're not overfeeding. Even if your child eats more than the kid next door, pediatricians normally don't consider diets or restrictions for infants or toddlers. There's considerable time for the correction of his body type through growth spurts and changes in eating habits over the first two to three years. And don't pay attention to those comments about your son. It's easy to be defensive, but remember that most remarks are made without ill will.

How early can a child be put on a diet?

While it's important to begin watching a child's growth and eating pattern in the school years, diets as we think of them shouldn't be emphasized. This is a period of tremendous growth when adequate calories and balanced nutrition are critical to a child's health and well-being. Joseph Piscatella, in his wonderful book *Fat-proof Your Child*, suggests that rather than consider restrictive diets that emphasize shape and physical appearance, the focus should instead be on healthy, balanced eating that fosters lifelong habits. This involves providing healthful food choices that emphasize what should be eaten as opposed to what shouldn't be eaten.

Restrictive diets do have a role in the management of the seriously obese child. However, these should be carefully prescribed and monitored by professionals experienced in pediatric weight management.

Our eleven-year-old son is significantly overweight at 125 pounds. What are the chances that he will be overweight as an adult?

Unfortunately, the chances are very good. Recent studies show that overweight children at this age have a 50 percent chance of being obese as adults as compared to nonobese children, whose chances are approximately 10 percent.

Defining a Weight Problem

While everyone has his or her own idea of how big is too big, obesity is medically defined based on a child's weight relative to her height. At any given height a child has an ideal weight, which, conveniently, is called the *ideal body weight* (IBW). Children who weigh 20 percent above their IBW are considered obese.

Another term you may see tossed around is the body mass index (BMI). The body mass index is another measure of body fatness. It is a useful index of obesity from age two through adulthood, and in childhood it predicts obesity in later adult life. It also tends to correlate well with the complications of obesity, such as high blood pressure and high cholesterol. BMI is calculated by dividing body weight in kilograms by the square of the height in meters (kg/m^2). Just like height and weight, BMI is plotted on a curve to obtain a percentile value. A child whose BMI plots between the eighty-fifth to ninety-fifth percentile is overweight. Above the ninety-fifth percentile a child is obese and at significant risk for obesity as an adult.

Despite the odds, there is still time for everyone to change. Everyone? Yes, everyone. Even if the child doesn't come from an obese family, successful pediatric obesity management programs dictate that the entire family should be involved in the child's recovery—much like an alcoholic. One child alone can't be expected to make the lifestyle changes necessary for weight loss and, most important, maintenance of healthy weight. Instead you, the parent, must commit to making lifestyle changes for the entire family to follow. Without a firm commitment to this at this age, the likelihood of your son becoming an obese adult is significant.

The Apple Doesn't Fall Far From the Tree

Do fat parents make kids who grow up to be fat adults? It appears that they do. A recent study in the *New England Journal of Medicine* found that parental obesity more than doubles the risk of adult obesity among both obese and nonobese children younger than ten years old. Prior to three years of age, the primary predictor of obesity in adulthood is a parent's obesity. Over the age of three, a child's obesity status begins to play more of a role in his or her ultimate obesity as an adult.

Our family doctor told us our son is twenty pounds overweight. He eats right and seems to exercise. Could this be genetic or perhaps a thyroid problem?

Genetic or metabolic problems are an exceptionally rare cause of excessive weight gain in children. While physicians hold out hope for families that their child's condition could somehow be an easily treatable medical problem, these tests are usually fruitless. However, obesity is an area of active research, and interesting new discoveries are uncovered every month. Various mutations and defects involving appetite control and fat metabolism have already proven that the more severe cases of obesity may have a strong genetic component. In the past we have looked on those with weight control issues as lazy or lacking self-control. While an individual's will may, in part, control his destiny, the role of the gene can't be ignored. It's very likely that in our lifetime

> **An Ounce of Prevention Is Worth a Pound (or Two) of Cure**
>
> Establishing healthful eating patterns and incorporating physical activity in your family's routine may be the best way to treat obesity. It can help the young children in the family maintain an appropriate body size and help those ample adults in the family trim up a little. A healthy lifestyle can be a great heirloom.

we'll see the discovery of correctable genetic defects that explain the seemingly unexplained paradox of your overweight child who seems to eat right and exercise.

As vegetarians, we would like to raise our son on a similar diet. Is it safe?

The suitability of any diet for a child depends on its ability to provide the proper amounts of energy, protein, and nutrients for normal growth and development. While your vegetarian diet may be a safe and healthy alternative for you, keep in mind that your baby has different nutritional needs.

One type of vegetarian diet that is unsafe for young children is the *vegan* diet, which excludes all foods of animal origin—meat, fish, eggs, and dairy products. Unless supplemented, this diet is deficient in vitamin B12 and calcium and over the long term can have serious consequences for the growing child. This diet also tends to be high in bulk but low in calories. So in order for a child to meet his daily caloric requirement, he would need to eat more to make up the difference. This can be a problem for babies and toddlers who have small stomachs and can be picky about their food selection. While a vegan child might get enough protein, consuming enough food to provide energy is probably the bigger obstacle. This problem usually can be overcome by changing to a less restrictive vegetarian diet.

For example, *lacto-ovo vegetarians* exclude meat, poultry, fish, and shellfish from their diet but will eat diary products and eggs. *Lacto-vegetarians* follow a similar diet but don't eat eggs. These diets allow you to offer your child a wide variety of foods such as cheese, butter, sour cream, and other dairy products that are valuable sources of calories.

Other high-calorie vegetarian foods include avocados, dates, nuts, and olives. Remember, fatty foods are the highest source of calories for the least intake, which is essential when feeding a toddler or baby.

Types of Vegetarians

While any individual may choose their degree of vegetarianism, the following represent the most commonly recognized "categories":

Semivegetarian: Allows dairy, eggs, seafood, and sometimes poultry; avoids red meat.

Lacto-ovo-vegetarian: Allows dairy products and eggs; avoids meat, poultry, fish, and seafood.

Lacto-vegetarian: Allows milk and milk products; avoids meat, poultry, eggs, and seafood.

Vegan: No animal products; avoids dairy, eggs, meat, seafood, and poultry

---

Is it better for children to eat their vegetables raw as opposed to cooked?

Since some of the nutrients found in vegetables may be lost with boiling, steaming, or microwaving, raw vegetables do have the nutritional edge. The effect, however, is not significant enough to warrant a raw-or-nothing approach. Certainly, during the first two to three years of life, vegetables like broccoli, carrots, zucchini, and squash must be cooked to be soft enough to eat. However they're prepared, any vegetable is better than none at all.

I've been criticized by my mother-in-law for serving canned and frozen vegetables to my daughter. She seems to think they're less nutritious. Is this true?

It sounds like your mother-in-law needs some updated nutrition information. Fresh vegetables aren't necessarily better than canned or frozen. Frozen and canned vegetables are processed immediately, locking in their nutrients. Fresh vegetables, on the other hand, can lose their nutritional potency during the weeks of storage and travel before sale. The nutritional differences among fresh, frozen, and canned vegetables are minimal. While some studies have found higher levels of iron and folate in canned veggies and more vitamin C in fresh and frozen, the differences aren't worth bickering about, especially with your mother-in-law. Serve vegetables in whatever form you feel most comfortable and in whatever form facilitates inclusion in your daughter's diet.

I've heard all sorts of things about the health benefits of soy protein. Does this apply to children?

Yes, the health benefits that adults enjoy from soy protein apply as well to children. A readily available and versatile food source, soy is a rich source of protein without the saturated fat of dairy, eggs, and meat. Consequently, the consistent use of soy has been shown to lower cholesterol levels and improve the balance of good to bad cholesterol. While the issue of saturated fat and cholesterol may not seem like a pressing issue for your child, there is evidence that the groundwork for arteriosclerosis is laid during childhood.

Soy also gets full marks as a source of iron and calcium. Considering that iron recently has been found to be one of the most deficient nutrients among American toddlers, this versatile protein source should be tried on every high chair.

And despite the fact that their effect on infants and children isn't fully understood, the presence of phytoestrogens may be considered a bonus. Phytoestrogens are naturally occurring hormonelike substances found in a variety of foods including apples, wheat, and soy. They are touted to offer potential therapy for a variety of conditions, from cancer to heart disease, although little scientific evidence exists to support their widespread clinical use. And among populations that maintain soy as a staple part of their diet, hormone-dependent cancers like prostate and breast cancer are known to occur less frequently.

While some of these benefits may seem too good to be true, soy protein represents a healthful alternative that probably can't hurt and likely will help.

Vegetarians: A Fact Sheet

How many? According to the U.S. Department of Agriculture, there are 7 million to 8 million self-declared vegetarians in the country today (about 2.5 percent of the populace).

Is this a youth movement? Increasingly, yes. A recent Roper Poll shows 8 percent of thirteen- to seventeen-year-olds eschewing meat (more than double the percentage for adults), while 11 percent of teen girls say they've sworn off meat.

Are the diets beneficial? In many ways, yes. Recent health studies show significantly reduced rates of heart disease and breast/prostate/colon cancer among adults who were vegetarian as children.

Do "veggie" children grow up as strong and healthy as "nonveggies"? Yes, provided they get all of the required micro-nutrients. A U.S. Centers for Disease Control study of 404 vegetarian children, published in *Pediatrics* (O'Connell J M, et al. "Growth of Vegetarian Children: the Farm Study." 1989; 84:475–81), found their growth patterns to be the same as those of nonvegetarians.

SOURCE: *AAP NEWS* (JUNE 1999).

HEALTHY HEARTS

Can children develop coronary artery disease?

While it has been shown that children begin to develop arteriosclerosis from an early age, significant recognizable disease is very rare. In cases where it is known to occur, it is associated with rare genetic disorders and inherited diseases of lipid metabolism.

When should children begin to follow a low-fat, heart-healthy diet?

Since fat and adequate calories are critical to the growing body and brain, it has been suggested that children be withheld from a low-fat diet until after the age of two. Between two and five years, a child can gradually start to assume a more adultlike balance of fat in her diet. By the start of the school years it is recommended that children should receive only 30 percent of their calories from fat just like adults.

Is it necessary for children to have their cholesterol levels checked?

While a controversial issue, most experts in pediatric nutrition don't recommend routine screening of children for cholesterol. How these values are interpreted in children and the best means of treating them are a matter of speculation since little research has been done in this area. Lipid screening should be a selective process for children from families at high risk for cardiovascular disease. This includes a family history of elevated blood lipid or heart attack before age fifty-five.

Children found to have blood lipid levels above acceptable values for their age are typically placed on a diet limiting their saturated fat intake to 10 percent of their calories. Review of follow-up blood levels done after three months of dietary restriction will determine whether further changes are necessary. While medications sometimes are used, most children are managed with diet.

Considering the importance of caloric intake in the growing child, close supervision by an experienced pediatric dietician is critical throughout this entire process. And depending on the degree of lipid disturbance in your child's blood, input may be necessary from a gastroenterologist, geneticist, or other specialist with expertise in inherited lipid disorders.

VITAMINS AND MINERALS

How do I know if my toddler needs a vitamin?

While the traditional teaching has been that if children follow a balanced diet, they'll get what they need, that may not be the case any longer. According to recent studies, approximately 50 percent of one- to two-year olds are not meeting their Reference Daily Intake (RDI) for iron and calcium and approximately 80 percent are missing their RDI for zinc and vitamin E. The statistics regarding iron are most worrisome since iron has been closely linked to mental and motor development.

Does this mean your toddler should be receiving a daily vitamin? Probably, since even among the best eaters it's impossible to know for sure if they're meeting their needs. Unfortunately, most liquid vitamin supplements marketed for one- to two-year-olds don't contain zinc. This can be addressed by providing half of a chewable vitamin intended for an older toddler. They tend to be crumbly and can be handled by most young toddlers with a little bit of water.

To complicate matters further, most vitamins for children in this age group contain no calcium. If your child is a good milk drinker, this shouldn't be a problem. Otherwise, a number of palatable foods represent good sources of calcium. In unusual cases where calcium is critical and we're faced with a child who refuses all major sources of this key nutrient, half of a chewable calcium-based antacid tablet does the trick. This should be administered only under the supervision of a pediatrician or a pediatric dietician.

Some Multivitamins Don't Contain Calcium

Don't count on your local children's vitamin to cover your child's calcium needs since most don't contain calcium. This is one of the frustrating shortcomings of supplemental vitamins and requires a creative approach to feeding. Look for a "complete" or "with calcium" version of your favorite chewable vitamin, and be sure to check the label.

If your child is a lousy milk drinker or is otherwise picky, other valuable sources of calcium include fortified orange juice, yogurt, cheese, blackstrap molasses, and dried apricots. Frozen waffles also represent an appealing option for picky toddlers, with each one packing 150 mg of calcium. Your pediatrician may consider recommending half of a chewable calcium-based antacid since this is a terrific way to meet a child's calcium needs.

How are "natural" vitamins different from regular vitamins?

There is no difference. A vitamin is a vitamin no matter how it's packaged. Vitamin C, for example, has one and only one molecular structure that's always the same, no matter where it comes from. While vitamins may be packaged in various ways, what you're getting in the final analysis is all the same.

Fact or Fiction: Vitamins Help Children Grow

Fiction. Parents often feel urgency about having their underweight child on vitamins with the belief that they will help them grow. While vitamins are critical to a variety of body functions, they do not directly initiate growth.

Is there really any rationale to providing different colors on a child's plate?

The rich and vibrant colors of fruits and vegetables reflect their nutrients, and a varied plate means a balance of those nutrients. Red and orange vegetables are rich in *lycopene* and *beta-carotene*, which have been found to have cancer-fighting properties. Dark-green vegetables also contain beta carotene in addition to *anthocyanin*, another anticancer pigment. In addition to the built-in nutrient value of these foods, a colorful presentation may impact on how it's received by a discriminating toddler.

Fact or Fiction: Eating Carrots Will Help Improve Your Eyesight

Fiction. While deficiency of vitamin A (a nutrient found in carrots in abundance) has been associated with night blindness, there's no evidence that carrots improve the vision of children with otherwise normal diets.

How do I know if my child is iron deficient?

Iron deficiency is a frequent concern among parents, and for good reason. Recently a significant number of American children have been found to be falling short on their dietary intake of iron. Since iron is one of the nutrients closely associated with long-term cognitive and motor development, parents and pediatricians must make sure that children receive their daily value for iron. This is easier said than done, however, since children who are reported to be excellent eaters are frequently deficient in nutrients such as iron.

So how will you know when there's a problem? In most cases you won't be able to tell based on how your child looks or what she does. In the early or mild cases of iron-deficiency anemia, the only way to detect a problem is through a blood count. Since iron is a key ingredient in hemoglobin, the oxygen-carrying chemical found in red blood cells, the first thing to change will be a child's blood count. Anemia, or a decrease in red blood cells, is the telltale sign of iron deficiency. Once iron-deficiency anemia becomes more severe, children may look pale or become easily fatigued.

If you have concerns about your child's iron intake or the possibility of iron deficiency, talk to your pediatrician. A simple blood test is all that's required to rule it out. And should your child fall short, the treatment is easy. In the event that your physician has concerns beyond a simple dietary deficiency, other tests may be considered to rule out sources of iron loss, such as blood in the stool.

Fact or Fiction: Eating Dirt Is a Sign of Iron Deficiency

Fact. Eating dirt, paper, and other nonfood items is a classic symptom of iron deficiency in children. This condition is referred to as *pica*. Iron-deficient adults often chew ice or crave crunchy food.

I have heard that there are different types of iron. Which one is best for my child?

Children get their iron from two major sources: meat and vegetables. The iron from these two dietary sources is absorbed differently. The iron found in animal tissue is called *heme iron*. Ten to twenty percent of heme iron is absorbable, making it one of the most richly absorbed dietary sources of this vital mineral. The *nonheme iron* found in vegetables and fortified food products is absorbed about a third less efficiently, at around 7 percent. While it may appear that meat is the way to go, it should be understood that both meat and vegetables play important roles in a balanced diet and the type of iron each contains shouldn't be a primary factor influencing food choice.

Why is iron best taken with vitamin C?

Iron is available in various forms and its absorption is dependent on what food it comes from. In addition to this, other factors, such as the food that is ingested with the iron, influences how it's absorbed. Vitamin C enhances iron absorption. It allows iron to reach the lining of the intestine in a form that's easier to transport into the blood. In addition to vitamin C, both citrate and animal protein (meat, fish, poultry) enhance the absorption of iron. It's also interesting to note that children who are iron deficient absorb iron more efficiently than those with normal iron status.

If it seems that iron is a sensitive element, you're right. Just as there are foods and vitamins that improve its absorption, so too are there those that inhibit its absorption. Tannins and phytates found in teas and certain vegetables bind iron and keep it from where it needs to go. Excessive calcium can inhibit the absorption of the iron found in meat.

So what should you do to help improve your child's chances of absorbing the iron she needs? In your day-to-day diet, common sense prevails. Given that the proteins found in meat improve the iron we take from our vegetables, serve a balanced plate. If your child is under treatment for iron deficiency, offer her iron supplement in between meals with a glass of orange juice or other vitamin C–containing drink.

Medically Speaking: Fortified vs. Enriched

If you read enough labels, you're bound to see "enriched" or "fortified" gracing the packages of your bread or cereal.

Enrichment restores essential nutrients that are lost during the processing of foods. Watch out for this one. When manufacturers have to put something back to make it as good as it was before, it usually means that the food is very processed.

Fortification describes the supplementation of important nutrients to food to make sure people get enough. An example is the addition of iron to cereal and vitamin D to milk.

Why are iron overdoses so dangerous for children?

Iron overdoses are an unfortunately common event in young families because expectant mothers often require prenatal iron and toddlers are always curious. As with any type of overdose, the danger of the medication is directly related to the amount taken. Moderate to severe iron overdoses in children may cause liver damage, low blood sugar, shock, and even coma. Since iron is irritating to the stomach even in normal doses, an overdose can lead to intestinal bleeding and ulcers. These ulcers and irritation have been known to lead to scarring and partial blockage of the stomach weeks after the ingestion. As with all medications, keep iron well out of the reach of children.

Iron-rich Foods
Liver
Red meat
Prunes, prune juice, and raisins
Pumpkin and sunflower seeds (not for children under two)
Watermelon
Wheat germ and bran
Iron-fortified cereals
Blackstrap molasses (not for children under two unless pasteurized)
Leafy green vegetables such as spinach and collard greens

Do vitamin C supplements help prevent illness in children?

Despite what we hear from the popular health movement, there is little evidence to support the idea that vitamin C decreases a child's susceptibility to bacterial or viral infections. Excessive or megadose treatments of vitamin C or any vitamin should never be used with children. Large doses of vitamin C have been associated with diarrhea, kidney stones, decreased absorption of vitamin B12, and copper deficiency.

My son doesn't eat much fruit.
Does he need a vitamin C supplement?

It's exceptionally rare that a child needs to take a vitamin C supplement. If it seems your child isn't interested in fruit, be sure that you've explored all of the colorful options that pack a vitamin C punch, such as strawberries, tomatoes, bell peppers, and citrus fruits. If your child still holds out, natural fruit juices, such as orange juice and vitamin C–fortified beverages, usually will do the trick. An eight-ounce glass of orange juice from concentrate contains 104 mg of vitamin C, which is well above the 45 mg recommended daily value for children ages four to ten years. Infants and toddlers need 20 to 30 mg per day.

Do zinc supplements help prevent colds?

There has been a recent flurry of media attention suggesting that zinc may be the antidote to the common cold. While zinc may be critical to infection-fighting white blood cells, there is no evidence to support its role treating viruses in children. A recent study appearing in the *Journal of the American Medical Association* found that cold symptoms didn't go away any sooner for children age six to eighteen who took a zinc lozenge compared with those taking a cherry placebo. To make matters worse, the children taking the zinc reported a bad taste in their mouths, diarrhea, nausea, and sore throat as side effects.

NOT SO NATURAL

Are snacks made with olestra safe for children?

Olestra is the latest move by the food industry to make us feel less guilty about eating junk. As an artificially produced fat that's affectionately known as sucrose polyester, olestra has the taste, consistency, appearance, and texture of triglyceride fat traditionally found in savory snacks. What's different is that olestra isn't absorbed and doesn't contribute to the calories and fat that we typically think about when we eat junk food. Instead, olestra makes it through our intestinal tract unscathed with no impact on our waistline or coronary arteries. Sounds pretty good so far? It is—except that early

---

Medically Speaking: RDA: What Is It Really?

Once established as a way to ensure good nutrition for military recruits, the RDA, or recommended daily allowance, has been replaced by the following terms:

Daily value (DV). Once the RDA, the DV replaces it and is made up of DRV and RDI.

Daily reference value (DRV). Provides guidelines for intake of protein, carbohydrates, fats, cholesterol, fiber, sodium, and potassium.

Reference daily intake (RDI). Provides guidelines for intake of essential vitamins and minerals.

Despite what terms the government chooses to use to describe what we should be eating, the most important thing to understand is what it really means. Daily values (old RDA) are established to cover what the average person should take to prevent any question of deficiency. In most cases, these are much more than what the average child needs for normal growth and development. As a public health standard, the daily value aims to cover the needs of the majority of the population, and it may not necessarily apply to any one person.

---

studies with this seemingly magic fat found that it interfered with the absorption of certain vitamins that depend on fat as part of the digestive process. Consequently, these vitamins are added back to foods containing olestra to make up for what may be lost through its use.

While this may seem risky for children because they are so dependent on their vitamins, there are no conclusive studies to suggest that olestra is harmful. As with most foods, just about anything in moderation is acceptable. If you allow olestra chips as frequently as you should allow any other type of savory snack (i.e., on occasion in limited amounts), there should be no concerns about its safety.

Does olestra cause diarrhea?

As a nonabsorbed fat, olestra has the potential to cause diarrhea when eaten in excess. Assuming that olestra-containing snacks are consumed in moderation, diarrhea shouldn't be a problem.

I have heard that Nutrasweet (aspartame) is unsafe for certain children. How do I know if my child is one of them?

Aspartame is an artificial sweetener commonly used in soft drinks and beverages. Aspartame is made up of two compounds, phenylalanine and aspartic acid, which are broken down in the body. Phenylalanine is normally broken down in the liver without a problem. Individuals with the genetic condition *phenylketonuria* (PKU) lack this ability to break down phenylalanine and accumulate it in the body when it is ingested. While this may not be much of an issue for adults with PKU, the developing brain is very sensitive to the effects of phenylalanine. Children with this disorder can sustain permanent injury when exposed to phenylalanine either in utero or early in life. Consequently, children with PKU can't take aspartame. PKU is tested for as part of a baby's routine newborn screening.

How old should a child be before allowing regular consumption of Nutrasweet?

There is no reason why aspartame shouldn't be safe for children of any age. While concerns have been raised about the possible effects of phenylalanine on a child's brain chemistry, there is nothing to support these theoretical claims. However, just because this particular artificial sweetener doesn't appear to be harmful doesn't mean that it has a role in a child's diet. Aspartame sweetens sodas and other beverages, which should have only a limited place in any child's diet. Milk, water and 100 percent juice should be the liquid staple for all children until well into their school-age years. At that point sodas and other sweetened drinks can take the coveted position of occasional treats.

What is genetically modified food?

Genetically modified (GM) food is food whose DNA has been altered through the introduction of genes from another organism. The idea is to integrate genes that provide some advantage to the plant, perhaps to withstand a colder climate or be more resistant to pests. While this has been done for years through cross-hybridization, a process where pollen from one plant is placed on another, genetic modification allows the introduction of genes from different species.

The use of genetically modified foods has raised concern among environmental groups although there's no evidence that they're unsafe for consumption. What's being produced or "expressed" in a genetically modified plant are typically proteins just like those we consume in our daily diets. In other cases, genes are used to prevent certain traits from being expressed. A great example of this is the Flavr-Savr tomato (Monsanto Company). In the Flavr-Savr tomato, one of the key enzymes responsible for tomato ripening and softening is inhibited. This results in a tomato with a much longer shelf life.

While the consumption of GM food may be harmless, the potential impact on the world's ecosystem may be a different story. One of the most controversial GM foods is bt corn, a genetically modified corn that contains a bacterial gene lethal to certain caterpillars. While most bt corn is used for animal feed, some is used to make the corn syrup frequently found in processed food. It has been found that the pollen from bt corn can kill monarch butterflies, which are part of the same class of insects that it's intended to target. As a result of consumer concerns over environmental and health concerns, farmers have been slowly turning away from the use of bioengineered corn. It represented 25 percent of the 1999 corn crop but only 19 percent of the 2000 crop.

Is organic food more nutritious than regular food?
By most standards the term "organic" implies that the food in question was raised without the use of artificial pesticides or fertilizers. According to the new national standards for organic food recently released by the U.S. Department of Agriculture, there are well-defined terms to describe the production, handling, and processing of organic food. Independent of how organic a food may be, these terms says nothing

about the actual nutritional value of the food. While food grown with limited use of pesticides and artificial fertilizers has obvious health benefits, organic and nonorganic foods should be equally nutritious.

How safe is monosodium glutamate (MSG) for children?

MSG, a compound derived from seaweed, has been a recognized flavor enhancer for nearly 100 years. MSG has been found to be safe for adults who consume less than 55 milligrams per day. While safe levels for children haven't been reported, moderation should be the rule, as with any type of processed food. Children with asthma should avoid MSG, since this is one of the few medical conditions that it has been found to aggravate.

My son enjoys canned macaroni with meat sauce. I recently looked at the nutrition label and found that one serving contains 900 mg of sodium. Is this healthy?

This is excessive sodium by any measure, and it isn't healthy. However, assuming that your child has normal kidneys and no other major medical problem that requires limited sodium,

---

How Organic Is Organic?

Until recently, the idea of what constituted organic food was debated among over forty different state and private agencies. Just in time to settle the debate, the U.S. Department of Agriculture has released standards for the production, handling, and labeling of organic foods. According to these new standards, any food labeled organic must be produced with a very limited number of pesticides and fertilizers and must not involve the use of ionizing radiation or genetic manipulation. Look for the following four categories of organic food:

100 percent organic. Consists entirely of organic ingredients.
Organic. Consists of at least 95 percent by weight organic ingredients.
Made with organic ingredients. Between 70 and 95 percent of the contents must be organic.
Product with less than 70 percent organic ingredients. As the name suggests, consists of less than 70 percent organic ingredients. Labeling of these products as organic must be limited to the ingredient panel and cannot involve the front of the package.

most children should be able to handle a meal like this without a problem. Despite the fact that it may do no harm from time to time, it shouldn't be habit. Childhood feeding patterns become adult eating habits, and the salt, sugar, and seasoning that we allow sets the pace for the long haul. Try your own macaroni with low-sodium tomato sauce and limit convenience meals in a can to once or twice a week.

What's the connection between attention deficit disorder and sugar intake?

Sugar and food additives have long taken the blame for hyperactivity in children. Despite this widely held belief, well-designed clinical studies have failed to show any connection between sugar intake and behavior (or misbehavior). On a similar note, studies looking at the Feingold diet, a diet that eliminates artificial colorings and flavorings to treat attention deficit hyperactivity disorder (ADHD), have failed to show any connection between additives and behavior.

How is it possible to distinguish between food poisoning and a virus?

Food poisoning is a phrase used to describe a number of bad things that can happen when you eat the wrong food from the wrong place. Tainted food causes illness through the proliferation of a bacterial organism in a child's digestive tract. An example would be an intestinal infection with the *Shigella* organism from contaminated chicken. In this case the bacteria multiplies in the colon and releases a toxin causing tissue damage and cramping. Other forms of illness are caused by toxins found in food and involve no infection. An example of this would be shellfish contaminated by the toxin associated with the red tide.

Given the various types of food contamination that we may be exposed to, poisoning can present itself in any number of ways, and it may be difficult to discern from a virus. The most common symptoms of foodborne illness are diarrhea, abdominal cramps, vomiting, head and muscle aches, and fever. Most symptoms appear twelve to seventy-two hours after eating the tainted food but may come on as early as thirty minutes after. Viruses tend also to be accompanied by fever and may include other symptoms such as rash or swollen glands. Foodborne illnesses often involve other members of the family in a very similar way with a very similar time course. Viruses, on the other hand, are likely to be passed from person to person, making everyone sick at slightly different times.

Children seriously ill from food poisoning almost always deserve medical attention. A physician may be able to discriminate between virus and food poisoning based on your child's story. While a stool sample may be able to identify a bacterial organism that may have taken up residence in your child's colon, most types of food poisoning due to toxins won't be able to be identified. Often we're faced with several members of a family or party all violently ill after eating the same thing with no evidence of infection or toxin. In these cases the local department of health may be able to identify the original source of the illness and in turn identify the type of contamination.

I've heard that the FDA has recently approved the use of radiation to sterilize food. How safe is this?

While the idea of irradiating food to keep it safe runs counter to the way most of us think, consider that the diseases associated with foodborne illness are responsible for hundreds of deaths and countless hospitalizations each year. Colitis-causing bacteria such as *E. coli* and *Shigella* are responsible for the fast food–associated outbreaks of diarrhea and the dreaded hemolytic uremic syndrome so often reported in the press. Prenatally acquired infections with organisms such as *Listeria* and *Toxoplasma* can cause miscarriage or severe brain injury with lifelong consequences. Medical expenses and job loss from foodborne illness account for some $5 to $23 billion per year.

Mommy, Can I Lick the Spoon?

Not so fast. Despite what your grandma let you do, licking the spoon should be taboo if there are eggs in the batter. Raw eggs can contain traces of the salmonella organism, which may cause a severe intestinal infection.

Food irradiation is designed to prevent all of this by briefly penetrating food and reducing the numbers of microorganisms that can naturally inhabit foods. While food irradiation has been used to treat foods such as fruit and dry spices, the U.S. Department of Agriculture (USDA) amended its food safety regulations in early 2000 to allow the use of ionizing radiation to treat uncooked meat and meat by-products. In addition to reducing the risk of exposure to pathogenic organisms, food irradiation extends shelf life, eliminates some pests, and potentially reduces the use of chemicals and other additives. This process also carries the advantage of allowing treatment of food after it has been completely sealed, thereby preventing subsequent contamination.

Concerning safety, neither the exposed food nor its packaging become radioactive during the process. Numerous studies on treated foods have failed to show any dangerous by-products, and taste is unaffected. Despite what the USDA deems safe, in the final analysis you'll have to weigh the remotely odd feeling of preparing a meal with irradiated meat against the remotely small risk of serving potentially tainted meat. No one said raising kids in the new millennium was going to be easy.

For more information on food irradiation, contact the Food Safety and Inspection Service of the USDA by phone at (202) 720-3897 or visit the website at *www.fsis.usda.gov/OA/topics/irrmenu.htm.*

How will I know if the meat I'm buying has been irradiated?
Irradiated meat and poultry products will require labeling with the international symbol of food irradiation, the radura. Products must state that they are "Treated by radiation."

What is bST?
BST is short for *bovine somatotropin,* or bovine growth hormone. bST is a protein hormone used in dairy cows to stimulate and improve the efficiency of milk production.

Is there any difference in the milk from bST supplemented cows and unsupplemented cows?

bST-stimulated milk is indistinguishable in taste, color, flavor, or nutrient content from nonstimulated milk, and the levels of bST are no different. It should be noted that bST stimulates the production of a protein called *IGF-1* in the cow, and these levels are higher when compared with nonsupplemented cows. IGF-1 is naturally found in both cow's milk and human milk, and it's broken down in the stomach and small intestine just like any other protein. As with any other naturally occurring protein or protein hormone that may make its way into our diet, IGF-1 has no activity when taken by mouth.

Since the milk from bST-stimulated cows is virtually indistinguishable from that from nonsupplemented cows, it is felt that this milk is safe for human consumption. Independent reviews by the National Institute of Health, the World Health Organization, and the Inspector General of the Department of Health and Human Services have concluded that the milk from bST supplemented cows can be safely consumed.

What can I do to help prevent food-related infections in my children?

Everyone should follow these four simple steps to food safety:

1. *Clean: Wash hands and surfaces often.*
   Bacteria, viruses, and parasites can be spread throughout the kitchen and get onto cutting boards, utensils, and countertops. Here's how to prevent contamination with these kitchen critters:

   - Wash your hands with hot, soapy water before and after handling food and after using the bathroom, changing diapers, and handling pets.
   - Wash your cutting boards, dishes, utensils, and countertops with hot, soapy water after preparing each food item and before you go on to the next food.
   - Important: Rinse raw produce in water. Don't use soap or detergents. If necessary, use a small vegetable brush to remove surface dirt.

2. *Separate: Don't cross-contaminate.*
Cross-contamination is the word for how bacteria, viruses, and parasites can be spread from one food product to another. This is especially true when handling raw meat, poultry, seafood, and eggs, so keep these foods and their juices away from ready-to-eat foods. Here's how to prevent cross-contamination:

- Separate raw meat, poultry, and seafood from other foods in your grocery shopping cart and in your refrigerator.
- If possible, use a different cutting board for raw meat, poultry, and seafood products.
- Always wash hands, cutting boards, dishes, and utensils with hot, soapy water after they come in contact with raw meat, poultry, seafood, and eggs.
- Use separate plates for cooked foods and raw foods.

3. *Cook: Cook to proper temperatures.*
Food safety experts agree that foods are properly cooked when they are heated for a long enough time and at a high enough temperature to kill the harmful pathogens that cause foodborne illness.

- Use a clean thermometer that measures the internal temperature of cooked food to make sure meat, poultry, and casseroles are cooked to the proper temperature.
- Cook eggs until the yolk and white are firm. If you use recipes in which eggs remain raw or only partially cooked, use pasteurized eggs.
- Fish should be opaque and flake easily with a fork.
- When cooking in a microwave oven, make sure there are no cold spots where pathogens can survive. For best results, cover food, stir, and rotate for even cooking. If there is no turntable, rotate the dish by hand once or twice during cooking.
- Bring sauces, soups, and gravy to a boil when reheating. Heat other leftovers thoroughly to at least 165°F.

4. *Chill: Refrigerate promptly.*
Refrigerate foods quickly because cold temperatures keep harmful pathogens from growing and multiplying.

So set your refrigerator no higher than 40°F and the freezer at 0°F. Check these temperatures occasionally with an appliance thermometer and follow these steps:

- Refrigerate or freeze perishables, prepared foods, and leftovers within two hours or sooner.
- Never defrost food at room temperature. Thaw food in the refrigerator, under cold running water, or in the microwave.
- Marinate foods in the refrigerator.
- Divide large amounts of leftovers into shallow containers for quick cooling in the refrigerator.
- Don't pack the refrigerator. Cool air must circulate to keep food safe.

Source: Adapted from the American Medical Association, Centers for Disease Control, Food and Drug Administration, and the U.S. Department of Agriculture, *"Diagnosis and Management of Foodborne Illnesses: A Primer for Physicians,"* January 2001.

Some Closing Thoughts

It seems that just as soon as parents figure out how to get their children to eat, their concerns evolve into what they're actually eating. Ultimately we come to realize that what they're eating will influence the adults they'll someday become. There is good reason for these concerns because more and more we're coming to understand that adult disease has its roots in childhood. The seeds of coronary artery disease appear to be planted in childhood, and the habits we instill determine how those seeds are cultivated. Obesity and all of its complications appear to be closely related to obesity in childhood. Obese children appear to grow to become obese adults. It's also no coincidence that obese children are born of obese parents. So it seems that our influence as role models has a significant role in what our children will become.

Parents have a huge responsibility raising children in the twenty-first century. And despite the conveniences of modern life, there's never been a time more difficult to feed and raise children. The availability of so many quick, unhealthful foods makes it easy to avoid the preparation of wholesome, healthful alternatives. Our lifestyle, which seems to grow more fast-paced, encourages the prepackaged, processed microwave diet that's now considered the norm. Where and how we intercept the cycle is the choice of each individual parent.

While we all have plans of living and eating better, our lifestyle changes can't be made too early. In almost every other aspect of raising children, we're willing to change and adjust our way of living to suit the needs of our kids. In fact, it's almost standard that once children become toddlers, we see parents become compulsive with their choice of words. We've all lived with the consequences of a slipped expletive in front of a two-year-old. This truth also applies to how we feed and take care of ourselves in front of our children. Everything you eat and how you eat is observed by your kids from a very early age. The details of how we feed ourselves, much like the details of our speech, will dictate how our children will ultimately feed, grow, and live as adults. The health of our next generation requires a commitment to take care of ourselves and serve as the ultimate role model for a healthy lifestyle. While as pediatricians we have always insisted that children are not small adults, we should always be thinking about the adults whom they'll one day become.

Selected References

Diagnosis and Management of Foodborne Illnesses: A Primer for Physicians. January 2001. American Medical Association, Centers for Disease Control, Food and Drug Administration, and the United States Department of Agriculture.

Coyle, R., and Messing, P. *Baby Let's Eat!* New York: Workman, 1987.

Dietz, W. H., and Stern L. *American Academy of Pediatrics Guide to Your Child's Nutrition*. New York: Villard, 1999.

Eiger, M. S., and Wendkos Olks, S. *The Complete Book of Breastfeeding*, 3rd ed. New York: Workman, 1999.

Ezzo, G., and Bucknam, R. *On Becoming Babywise*. Sisters, Oregon: Multinomah Publishers, 1998.

Hendricks, K. M., Duggan, C., and Walker, W. A. *Manual of Pediatric Nutrition*, 3rd ed. London: B. C. Decker, 2000.

Huggins, K. *The Nursing Mother's Companion*, 4th ed. Boston: Harvard Common Press, 1999.

Kleinman, R. E. *Pediatric Nutrition Handbook*, 4th ed. Elk Grove Village, Illinois: American Academy of Pediatrics, 1998.

Kleinman, R. E., Jenninek, M. S., and Houston, J. *What Should I Feed My Kids?—The Pediatrician's Guide to Safe and Healthy Food and Growth*. New York: Fawcett, 1998.

LaForge, A. E. *Child Magazine's Guide to Eating*. New York: Pocket Books, 1997.

Martin, C. *The Nursing Mother's Problem Solver*. New York: Fireside, 2000.

Moll, L. *The Vegetarian Child—A Complete Guide for Parents*. New York: Perigee, 1997.

Neifert, M. *Dr. Mom's Guide to Breastfeeding*. New York: Plume, 1998.

Nissenberg, S. K., Bogle, M. L., Langholz, E. P., and Wright, A. C. *How Should I Feed My Child?* Minneapolis: Chronimed, 1993.

Pescatore, F. *Feed Your Kids Well*. New York: John Wiley, 1998.

Piscatella, J. C. *Fat-proof Your Child*. New York: Workman, 1997.

Roberts, S. B., Heyman, M. B., and Tracy, L. *Feeding Your Child for Lifelong Health*. New York: Bantam, 1999.

Rosenfeld, A., and Wise, N. *Hyper-parenting—Are You Hurting Your Child by Trying Too Hard?* New York: St. Martin's Press, 2000.

Satter, E. *Child of Mine—Feeding with Love and Good Sense*. Palo Alto; California: Bull Publishing, 2000.

Sears, W., and Sears, M. *The Family Nutrition Book*. New York: Little, Brown, 1999.

Shevlov, S. P. *Caring for Your Baby and Young Child—Birth to Age 5*. New York: Bantam, 1991.

Swinney, B. *Healthy Food for Healthy Kids*. New York: Meadow-book Press, 1999.

Tamborlane, W. V., ed. *The Yale Guide to Children's Nutrition*. New Haven, Connecticut: Yale University Press, 1997.

Wilkoff, W. G. *Coping with a Picky Eater*. New York: Fireside, 1998.

Yaron, R. *Super Baby Food*. Archbald, Pennsylvania: F. J. Roberts Publishing Co., 1998.

Index